The Moss Report - Endometrial Cancer Treatment Guide

Ralph W. Moss, PhD

Published by
The Moss Report
Stamford, CT
info@themossreport.com
https://www.themossreport.com/

ISBN for Paperback: 978-1-881025-41-2
ISBN for eBook: 978-1-881025-89-4

THE MOSS REPORT
themossreport.com

TABLE OF CONTENTS

APPENDICES

INTRODUCTION

The Moss Report was founded in 1974 by the medical science writer Ralph W. Moss, PhD, and is an independent information service offering critical views of conventional oncology and cancer treatment. Dr. Moss is widely considered the world's leading writer on complementary, integrative and alternative approaches and has been reporting on the state of cancer treatment since his time at Memorial Sloan-Kettering Cancer Center in New York City in the mid-1970s.

An essential feature of Dr. Moss' 50-year career is that his approach has never been promotional, but factual and pragmatic. It is not our intent to persuade you for or against any particular course of action. Rather, we carefully research each topic and then share what our deep dive into science has shown us. Decades of experience have taught us that the best results are obtained by people who integrate different approaches (both conventional and nonconventional) and, by doing so, attack cancer from various directions.

While the responsibility for treatment falls primarily in the hands of qualified oncologists and medical practitioners, we believe there is an essential self-help dimension to treatment as well. Collectively, *The Moss Report* resources offer a comprehensive and informed perspective for navigating the complexities of cancer care and treatment.

This *Cancer Treatment Guide* provides important general information concerning conventional treatments for cancer as well as a focus on the specific type of cancer. Although it is a standalone guide, it is designed to be used in conjunction with our companion book, *The Moss Method: Fight Cancer Naturally* and the resources on *The Moss Report* website.

What is in this Guide

- **Overview of the Cancer:** Details about its various types and key statistics.
- **Causes and Prevention:** Insight into how the cancer may develop and steps for its prevention.
- **Detection and Diagnosis:** Information on diagnostic procedures and what they mean for you.
- **Standard Treatments by Stage:** An outline of conventional treatment options, broken down by the stage of the cancer in question.
- **Implications of Treatments:** A discussion on what to expect from suggested treatments, including potential side effects (adverse events).
- **Evidence-Based Medicine:** Insight that will help you communicate better with your healthcare team.
- **Clinical Trials:** A look at their role in cancer research and innovation.
- **Additional Resources:** Where to find more information, including trusted publications and support networks.
- ***The Moss Method™*:** An introduction to Dr. Moss' nontoxic approach to fighting cancer naturally which is fully presented in our companion book, *The Moss Method: Fight Cancer Naturally*.

The purpose of this *Cancer Treatment Guide* in combination with *The Moss Method: Fight Cancer Naturally* and themossreport.com, is to help you find the optimal treatment plan for the particular cancer you are dealing with, whatever the stage.

A LETTER FROM RALPH W. MOSS, PHD

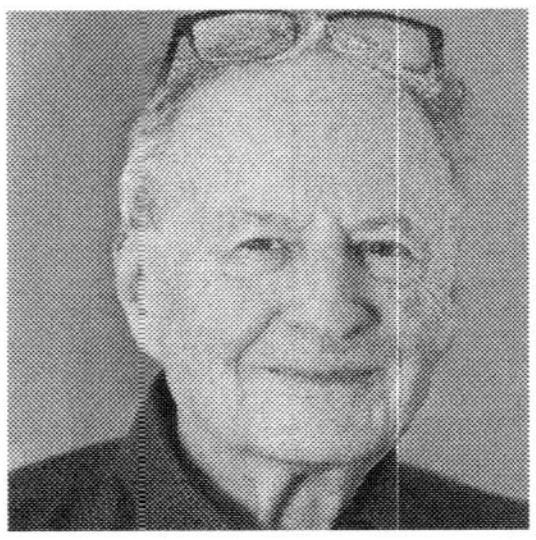

Dear Friend,

I want to extend a warm welcome to you from *The Moss Report*. For 50 years, it has been my mission to educate and empower cancer patients through the presentation of accurate information in terms that are readily understandable to lay people. I am honored to now be part of your healing journey.

Over the years, my thinking about cancer has evolved considerably. This is in line with the evolution of scientists' understanding of the disease, which is simply light years ahead of where it was half a century ago. I would like to share with you some of the core beliefs I have developed about cancer and the recovery process.

First, I believe in **integrative cancer care**. This means the skillful blending of conventional modalities (such as surgery, radiation and chemotherapy) with the broad field of complementary and alternative medicine (CAM). When I began my engagement in this field, there were two sharply delineated forms of cancer treatment: conventional and alternative. Conventional oncology consisted almost entirely of surgery, radiation, and chemotherapy. Alternative medicine was everything else.

Over time, especially after the founding of the complementary medicine department at the National Institutes of Health (NIH) of which I was a founding advisor, attitudes began to change. Today, the annual budget for the National Center for Complementary and Integrative Health is an extraordinary $170.3 million (FY 2023). The greatest triumph in this regard is the ascendancy of **immunotherapy**, the treatment of disease with substances that stimulate the immune response. Once in the realm of quackery, immunotherapy is now the undisputed fourth modality in cancer treatment.

I could also mention other treatments that have made the difficult transition from the fringe to the mainstream over the past 50 years:

- **Hyperthermia** or heat therapy (such as HIPEC for ovarian cancer).
- **Dietary modification:** Once the realm of "food faddists," today, it's well-established that certain dietary components and physical activity can play a role in cancer prevention, recurrence, and overall patient well-being.
- **High-dose intravenous vitamin C:** Once derided as useless, this has been shown in clinical trials at the University of Iowa to benefit cancer patients.
- **Targeted Therapies:** The idea of specifically targeting cancer cells without harming normal cells was a futuristic concept in the 1970s. With advances in molecular biology, today we have numerous targeted therapies, such as tyrosine kinase inhibitors, used routinely for many forms of cancer.
- **Cryotherapy:** Using cold to destroy tumors was an early idea that has now seen applications in certain localized cancers, such as prostate and cervical cancers. This was how my own prostate cancer was treated successfully at New York University Langone hospital in 2014.

There is hope that in the coming years, other forms of erstwhile "alternative medicine" will join the ranks of evidence-based treatments widely used at highly ranked hospitals in the U.S. and abroad.

Ideally, this melding of conventional and alternative therapies will take place within a single center of excellence, as was the case when I was treated at NYU's Langone's Department of Urology, now ranked #3 of all urology departments in the U.S. Finding this melding within one center, however, is rare today. Understanding this, one should seek to create a team in which each individual contributes to a combined approach and a better outcome. Conventional cancer treatments should be utilized when they have a proven track record of success and the fewest possible side effects. That said, I also believe there are scientifically valid treatments that come from outside conventional Western medicine. Let me demonstrate that with the story of my own encounter with prostate cancer.

My Cancer Journey

I had been writing about cancer for over 40 years when I myself was diagnosed with the disease. This happened in the summer of 2015. My wife and I had taken an unconventional blood test that could tell not only if you had cancer, but the specific type. (Sadly, that test is no longer available.) My wife's results were fine; but I scored positive for prostate cancer. But when I took these results to my urologist, she was skeptical. In fact, she assured me, "I am 100 percent certain you do not have aggressive prostate cancer!"

My Prostate Specific Antigen (PSA) test at that time had risen to 6.57 ng/mL (a normal score is 4.0 or lower) and my "free PSA" score had also edged into dangerous territory. But I had had somewhat elevated scores for 30 years. So she ascribed this to chronic prostatitis (inflammation of the prostate). Finally, at my urging, she agreed to write a prescription for a Magnetic Resonance Imaging (MRI) exam. I had done my homework and I insisted on having the latest "3T" scan. But this was not available in our town, and so my wife and I drove 200 miles to the nearest such facility. This was a famous university cancer center on the East Coast.

By then I was convinced that, at worst, the MRI would show a small focus of abnormal cells, which doctors call "prostatic intraepithelial neoplasia" (PIN). But, as fate would have it, the MRI showed the opposite: two large tumors in my prostate gland.

The next step was nearly disastrous. Of course, I needed to see a urologic oncologist immediately. Because we had traveled so far, the university hospital in question squeezed us in as the last scheduled appointment that Friday afternoon. This is never a good idea. Studies show that doctors "wear down" in the course of a day or a week, and, as a result, they may make inappropriate recommendations. There is even a name for this problem: "Decision Fatigue." One doctor has said: "The potential for complete decision exhaustion is astronomical."

(Linder JA, Doctor JN, Friedberg MW, et al. Time of day and the decision to prescribe antibiotics. JAMA Intern Med. 2014 Dec;174(12):2029-31) (https://blogs.jwatch.org/frontlines-clinical-medicine/2016/10/19/fighting-decision-fatigue/)

That Friday, the urologist in question slunk into the room, mumbled his last name by way of introduction, and, without making eye contact, sat down at the computer terminal and began fumbling with the keys. I had the sinking feeling that this weary middle-aged man could not wait to be done with his work week—and with me, his final patient.

He pulled up some records on the screen and looked over the radiologist's written summary of the MRI. After a minute, he blurted out words to this effect, "You've got a prostate full of cancer. It's broken through the capsule." These carelessly uttered words came as an indescribable shock to my wife and me. "Escaping the capsule" is the most critical question about any man's prostate cancer. But our own reading of the radiologist's report did not prepare us for the idea that this had happened. At that moment, I began to doubt my own interpretation. After all, radiologists write in highly technical jargon all their own. I have been reading such reports for about 40 years and make my living by translating 'Medicalese' into plain English. But when the patient is you, I discovered, it's a different story.

Confused, I asked the urologist to put the scans themselves up on the screen and show my wife and me where and how the tumors had compromised the capsule. His reaction was totally unexpected. He yelled, in anger and frustration, "I'm a urologist, not a radiologist! I don't analyze MRIs. I rely on the radiologists' reports."

He then suggested a biopsy, which he said could be arranged for early the next week. The doctor who would be doing the biopsy was the chairman of the department. I knew this because there was a poster in the waiting room announcing his retirement dinner.

I asked whether or not they would do a fusion biopsy, in which the MRI images were fused with live-time ultrasound to yield a more accurate sampling of the gland. No, we don't have that, was the curt reply. When I asked why, he said, "We can't afford it." I thought this was strange, since the hospital had just installed a Proton Therapy Center that cost $140 million. Then he rattled off the names of various nearby centers that did have this advanced technique, as if inviting me to go anywhere other than his clinic.

The only treatment he could suggest for my condition was radiation therapy since, as he claimed, my cancer was too far advanced for surgery. When I asked about my chances of being left impotent and/or incontinent after treatment, he exclaimed, "One hundred percent!"

That night, sitting on the edge of the bed in my hotel room, I called my friend, Geo Espinosa, ND. Geo is unique: a naturopathic doctor in the Department of Urology at Langone New York University (NYU) Medical Center. He strongly urged me to cancel the biopsy appointment that I had made and get a second opinion. So a few weeks later, I was in the New York City office of Samir Taneja, MD. Dr. Taneja had no problem taking my wife and me through the relevant online MRI images. Later, he performed a fusion biopsy. The good news: there was no indication that the cancer had pushed outside the capsule. That had been a complete and almost tragic mistake. (The thought has occurred to me that the first doctor was looking at the wrong patient's file.) I was in fact a candidate for curative treatment.

But the bad news was that my cancer, upon biopsy, was classified as a Gleason 8—high grade, poorly differentiated and aggressive. At this point, the textbook recommendations would be for surgery or intensive radiation therapy. But Dr. Taneja offered me another alternative: to ablate my tumors. Ablation means the destruction of cancer through nonsurgical and non radiological means. There are various ways of doing this. But what he suggested was cryoablation through the insertion of thin, cold probes. This would destroy just the tumors and a surrounding margin of normal cells, but it would spare most of the non-cancerous tissue. The normal portion of my prostate would be left intact and some of the crucial nerves would be spared.

So this is what I chose. The procedure was performed on an outpatient basis and was fully paid for by my health insurance. My costs involved staying in New York City for a few days. A day after the procedure I felt well enough to walk 20 blocks from our hotel to Greenwich Village. Most importantly, I soon had no lingering side effects from the treatment. And, without getting too graphic, some previous symptoms also improved.

All this happened more than eight years ago. At the one-year mark I had a follow-up biopsy and each year I go to New York for a follow-up 3T MRI. I am monitored with a complete PSA panel twice per year. All of my subsequent tests have been normal. Dr. Taneja is optimistic about my prospects, and of course I am very grateful for the excellent care I received at NYU. Naturally, I also employ select food supplements and have stepped up my dietary and exercise regimen to enhance the effect of this unusual innovative treatment.

My personal encounter with cancer has made me more aware of what many of my readers and consultation clients are going through on their own journeys. After 45 years in the field, I know a lot about cancer intellectually. But it is another thing to experience cancer on a personal and emotional level. So, while one never would choose to have cancer, it can pay dividends in terms of greater understanding and compassion.

Freedom of Choice

Many patients today are ready to assert their medical freedom of choice, are proactive regarding cutting edge treatments, and want to at least be involved in directing their own care. This does not mean eliminating medical practitioners from the decision-making process, but it does mean keeping ultimate control over decision-making. Older doctors, or those with a more authoritarian attitude, may still adhere to a "doctor knows best" model of care. But most doctors today are comfortable sharing ultimate responsibility, especially with well-informed patients and family members.

I also believe that reversing cancer and remaining well is more than just a physical process. Of course, aggressive medical treatments, such as surgery, radiation and chemotherapy, as well as less invasive therapies, have a central place in the treatment of this disease, and you need reliable and comprehensible information to make rational decisions about them. But there is another dimension to the cancer problem. As one long-term survivor put it:

"Returning to a state of health is not just about having treatment; it means dealing with the mental, emotional and the spiritual issues that tend to manifest physically. It means asking, 'Am I on the path that I want to be on?"

Some psychological after-effects are unavoidable. Getting a cancer diagnosis itself can be a trauma. For instance, there is the deplorable practice of comparing any horrible situation to cancer. It is difficult to wipe out such persistent cultural attitudes in a few years. The word "cancer" still strikes fear into us. Add to that, the fact that doctors are themselves all-too-human, but we tend to invest them with super-human qualities of omniscience and omnipotence. A careless word from a specialist—which may not reflect the actual state of affairs—can keep reverberating in your brain long afterwards. For that reason, I believe that many cancer patients are suffering from a type of post-traumatic stress disorder (PTSD). We talk glibly about the "war" on cancer, but as in other wars, the combatants and bystanders may pay the price for years afterwards.

This guide, along with the resources on our website and *The Moss Method: Fight Cancer Naturally*, is dedicated to helping you repair the mental and physical breach that cancer may have created in your life. To fully heal, you may need emotional healing as well. While it is easier to prescribe remedies for the body than the "soul", the attention you give these less tangible areas can speed the healing process and round out the effectiveness of your physical treatments. It can also serve as a profound source of strength, peace, and inspiration for you. Body, mind, and spirit are interwoven strands that form the whole person. In other words, approach healing holistically.

Another foundational understanding I hope to instill is that while I realize that on an emotional level many people still react to a diagnosis of cancer as a death sentence, one should resist any foregone conclusion. The attitudes of oncologists, family members, and friends may sometimes reinforce this kind of fatalistic notion. Doctors occasionally still deliver statistical averages of treatment effectiveness and survival as a certainty (often based on old and no-longer-valid statistics). In other words, you may hear "the disease is incurable," or "you have three, six or twelve months to live." The doctor may be trying to be accurate and to avoid giving false hope. Yet the result of such statements can be devastating to the patient. There is a strong societal drive to correct this sort of fatalism. I have my differences with the "cancer establishment", but this is one area in which they have done a very good job of trying to change fatalistic attitudes and 'normalize' cancer. This presents as less aggressive treatments (in general) and an improving situation in regard to the treatment of some advanced cancers.

In the past, at least, the typical "six months to live" speech could become a self-fulfilling prophecy. Some patients went into a tailspin, in a process that Harvard physiologist Walter Cannon, MD, called "voodoo death." In this case, on an emotional or subconscious level, patients became convinced that their situation was hopeless, which then contributed to their demise. It was and is hard to "un-hear" such dire predictions.
(Cannon WB. "Voodoo" death. Am J Public Health. 2002;92:1593-6; Lester D. Voodoo death. Omega (Westport) 2009;59:1-18)

In truth, one cannot know in advance how long any individual patient is going to live. That's called playing God. But this sort of fatalism is rapidly declining, as a group of younger and more socially diverse oncologists display a greater sensitivity to their patients' needs and feelings.

In War and Peace, Leo Tolstoy wrote in reference to his character Natasha's illness:

"Every living person has his own peculiar, personal, novel complicated disease unknown to medicine—not a disease of the lungs, liver, skin, heart and so on, mentioned in medical books, but a disease consisting of one of the innumerable combinations of maladies of those organs" (ch. 16).

A British physician named Thomas Lewis once wrote: *"Diagnosis is a system of more-or-less accurate guessing, in which the end-point achieved is a name. These names applied to disease come to assume the importance of specific entities, whereas they are for the most part no more than insecure and temporary conceptions. Even the various diagnostic categories of cancer are man-made constructs that mask the uniqueness of each individual's condition. Each person's cancer is only similar to, but not identical with, that of any other person with the 'same' diagnosis."*
(Lewis, Thomas. Reflections upon reform in medical education. The Lancet 1944;243(6298):619-621.)

So, after assimilating the facts of your disease, put aside the statistics. Defy the odds if it seems the best course for your treatment. Work in an optimistic way to heal yourself, body, mind, and spirit.

If names are "temporary conceptions," as Thomas Lewis said, then so too are predictions that are based on them. Never forget that **statistics are just averages**, not judgments of what must happen to you as a cancer patient. As one recovered patient wrote me:

"Remember, people aren't statistics. Statistics are made of people. Anybody can be the exception. It takes a while for others to be confident in your wellness but it must start with your own confidence in yourself and your own will to live, no matter what it takes. It isn't always easy. I am just now accepting that I am going to live in the long term. My doctors are becoming more confident, too!"

Bill's Story

Even very dire prognoses have their exceptions. Throughout the years, I have seen people survive the most threatening kinds of cancer, people whose chances, statistically speaking, seemed to be nil. Sometimes these "exceptional patients" used various unusual treatments. But on occasion, they did nothing special. Some years ago, my client and friend, Bill F., was diagnosed with colon cancer. When his cancer recurred after surgery and chemotherapy, Bill chose a treatment path that included yoga and herbal medicine. He not only survived years longer than expected, but lived his life to the full. Towards the end of his life he and his family went trekking in the mountains of Patagonia—something he had always wanted to do, but had deferred in his busy life.

Bill died on January 2, 2002, at the age of 66, seven years after his initial diagnosis. What made his case unusual was that in his professional life he was **William R. Fair, MD,** the esteemed chairman of the Urology Department at Memorial Sloan-Kettering Cancer Center (MSKCC) in New York City. He had been a conventional oncologist, who mocked "touchy feely" approaches, until personal experiences made him a passionate and outspoken advocate for the incorporation of non-conventional aspects of care. (http://www.nytimes.com/2002/01/13/nyregion/dr-william-fair-dies-at-66-an-expert-on-prostate-cancer.html)

Among other experiences, my friendship with Bill Fair made me a believer that there is a healing power inside us that is accessible to most of us. However, it is a real test of one's fortitude and conception of life. The body does have an inherent ability (which the ancients called the *vis medicatrix naturae*) to overcome disease and regain its equilibrium. This can provide a powerful underpinning to modern medicine. But ultimately you must find a way to activate that force.
(Neuburger, M. An historical survey of the concept of nature from a medical viewpoint. Isis. 1944;35:16–28)

In fact many of the treatments that I write about in this report (such as immunotherapy) are actually sophisticated ways of summoning up this self-healing power and bringing it into play in the fight against cancer. A relatively new class of drugs, called "immune checkpoint inhibitors," help free up the immune system. But it still takes a vigorous reaction on the part of the white blood cells to use that newly liberated system to attack and destroy the cancer. There is ample scientific evidence that shows that the mind, or psyche, is intimately involved in activating and 'motivating' the immune system to do just that.
(Hulett, Jennifer M., and Jane M. Armer. A systematic review of spiritually based interventions and psychoneuroimmunological outcomes in breast cancer survivorship. Integrative Cancer Therapies, 2016 Dec;15(4):405-423. Epub 2016 May 4.)

Please do not take any negative statistics to heart. Reject the "average patient" illusion that lies at their core. Let hope burn brightly within you! As the Roman philosopher Seneca once said, *"To wish to be cured is itself part of the cure" (pars sanitatis velle sanari fuit).*

Hope is the antidote to the psychological trauma engendered by the physical diagnosis. Hope is a tremendous force for healing. In 1859, the English poet Samuel Taylor Coleridge said, "He is the best physician who is the most ingenious inspirer of hope." He was talking about neurological problems, but the same holds true for cancer. With *The Moss Report*, you have information that can help you move forward towards hope and wholeness. But information alone is not enough. You must try to cultivate supporters and engage practitioners who share this belief, treat you with love and respect and radiate optimism. It is my personal belief that the main reason so many patients are turning towards complementary and alternative medicine (CAM) is because sometimes their more conventional doctors are themselves lacking in hope.

But, that said, there is hope. The purpose of *The Moss Report* is to unite hope with realism, the emotional and rational minds, by pointing you in the direction of scientifically credible and ethically defensible treatments. Commit yourself to an overall plan that nourishes your body, mind, and spirit. Be patient with yourself and the process, and reach out for help whenever you need it. Look for opportunities to replace negative beliefs, relationships and environments with more positive, life-affirming ones. This can be intense and difficult work. I feel it is important to adapt your techniques to the best resources that are available in your community and to your own spiritual orientation.

I have also seen many people use the crisis of cancer as a wake-up call. Rev. Clifford Oden once wrote a book titled *Thank God I Have Cancer*. A strange idea, but he was blessing the disease's transformative power. The celebrated physician-author Bernie Siegel, MD, reported that many patients say that cancer has been a very good thing in their lives. Similarly, the psychiatrist Lawrence LeShan, MD, praised cancer as a potential *"turning point"* in his famous book *Cancer as a Turning Point*. While I know that cancer is never a wished-for diagnosis, many people have found that the experience has helped them to settle difficult personal relationships, lead to the healing of old emotional wounds, and develop a deeper appreciation for the mysteries of existence. I hope this can be true for you as well.

I have found that patients are often paralyzed by fear, or exhausted by "battle fatigue" from their struggle. This is especially true with cancers that follow a protracted course. Patients may become confused by the many competing claims and systems (conventional Western, Ayurvedic, and Traditional Chinese Medicine, to name a few). Each has its own distinctive approach towards disease, including cancer. While it is wonderful to have access to options, it can open a Pandora's box of confusing claims and counterclaims. This "paralysis by analysis," as one client called it, is accentuated by the endless choices available over the Internet.

Your doctor may claim one thing, your acupuncturist another, and this report (or other things you have heard or read) even more. Whom should you believe?

The differences may be more of perspective than of facts. After all, conventional Western doctors have access to most of the same information I do. Over all, I see progress towards an integrative approach, even in the United States. We are moving towards a time of greater communication, cooperation, and respect among the various healing traditions. I believe that the work of the U.S. government's National Center for Complementary and Integrative Health (NCCIH), and of some individuals at the National Cancer Institute (NCI), has contributed to creating a more pluralistic medical culture called Integrative Oncology. However, differences still exist. If you experience a conflict between what others (such as your oncologists) have told you and what you read in thisreport or elsewhere, I urge you to probe more deeply. This is one of the main reasons that I give scientific references for most of my statements. I encourage you to further investigate these medical articles and to share this information with your doctors.

Ultimately, after intelligently assessing your options, you need to make treatment decisions. All my life I have promoted rational choices, yet in the end your choice may also involve a leap of faith. Knowing which treatment (and doctor) to choose requires using your intuition—your gut—as well as factual information.

Over the ancient Oracle at Delphi was engraved this simple prescription: *"Know Thyself."* In modern terms, "Know Thyself" means putting self-knowledge—including self-love—at the center of your decision-making process. Remember that beliefs themselves are powerful things, and believing in the treatments you choose is an important part of the healing process. This is as true of radiation or chemotherapy as it is of unconventional therapies. You have your own unique way of taking that leap with greater confidence. I hope this report will be helpful to you in choosing your unique path.

Albert Einstein told us: *"Imagination is more important than knowledge."* Einstein, the greatest scientist of the past century, told us that while research is important, we should trust our hearts. It is my ardent wish that you engage both science and personal feelings to embrace the healing path that is opening up before you. I believe this will give you the greatest possibility of a cure.

Sincerely,

Ralph W. Moss, PhD

A Couple of Notes

A note on quotations: I have taken the liberty of slightly altering some quotations to make for greater readability for lay persons. This includes sometimes putting words in bold or italics to highlight a point. But care has been taken not to alter the original intent.

A note on point of view: In this report, you'll find sections penned directly by me, Dr. Ralph W. Moss, where I express in the first person my analyses and perspectives. There are also segments where the voice represents *The Moss Report* as a collective entity. Both narrative styles interweave to offer a comprehensive understanding throughout.

On Statistics

It is important to understand that most of the response and survival figures that I cite in *The Moss Report Treatment Guides* come from standard medical sources. These refer to patients who primarily rely upon conventional treatments prescribed by academic and drug-oriented oncologists. Some of these figures are daunting. But I am optimistic that the best complementary and alternative (CAM) treatments can be integrated into conventional care. These can have a significant impact on both quality of life and overall survival.

Abbreviations

Note: Certain abbreviations are commonly used throughout this report:

- CAM = complementary and alternative medicine
- cm = centimeter, which equals 0.39 inches
- Et al. (Latin: et alii) = and others; it is used to complete a list, especially of other authors of a published work. In this report, I often refer to the first author when citing a work.
- When I refer to something appearing in "the literature," I am referring to the published, peer-reviewed scientific literature, such as one finds indexed in the PubMed database of 28 million articles or at www.asco.org. I will frequently cite these resources and strongly encourage you to use them as well. (http://www.ncbi.nlm.nih.gov/entrez/query.fcgi; one can just type in pubmed.com and it will redirect you there.)
- JAMA= Journal of the American Medical Association
- NCI = National Cancer Institute, the U.S. government's cancer research arm
- NIH = National Institutes of Health (parent organization of the NCI)
- QOL = quality of life
- ® = Registered commercial products are indicated with this symbol, but usually only for their first appearance in this report. We also do not always distinguish between registration (®) and trademark (TM).
- Drugs almost always have both a scientific name and one or more trade names. The scientific name is assigned by the Food and Drug Administration, while the trade name is proposed by the marketing company and approved by FDA. It is traditional in science

to refer to drugs by their scientific names, because trade names can vary by time and place. I generally provide both names, with the trade name in parentheses.

- The symbol "~" before a number means "approximately"
- WBH = whole body hyperthermia
- RCT = randomized controlled trial, the "gold standard" of clinical trials. Patients are randomly directed by computer to one or another treatment groups, in order to eliminate possible bias in the assignment of patients. Sometimes one of the treatment groups receives an inactive "dummy" medication called a placebo (from the Latin for "I shall please").

UNDERSTANDING CANCER

GENERAL INFORMATION ABOUT CANCER

Cancers in general share important characteristics: *cancer stem cells (CSCs)* have been found in almost every cancer type, the metabolism of most cancers is nearly identical, and the *immune system* is involved in almost every type and subvariety.

We understand that you are mainly interested in your particular cancer type. But it is important to also read about other cancers.

What we mean is, it is natural to focus on a particular cancer when seeking information. By doing so, however, it might limit your focus. For example, one may limit their search not just to breast cancer, but to, say, ER-positive, PR-positive, HER2-negative, breast cancer. By doing so, one can miss the forest for the trees.

In this guide, we drill down into the particulars of each cancer, but we also never lose sight of the bigger picture.

THE HALLMARKS OF CANCER: BACKGROUND, DEFINITIONS AND TREATMENT IMPLICATIONS

The fundamental question: **What is cancer?** I will share with you how almost all scientists now view this question. If you want to fully understand cancer from a different perspective, however, you need to read Prof. Thomas Seyfried's thought-provoking book, *Cancer as a Metabolic Disease*.

Most 21st century cancer research is grounded in the conceptual framework spelled out by Profs. Douglas Hanahan, of the Swiss Institute for Experimental Cancer Research (ISREC), Lausanne, and Robert A. Weinberg, of the Massachusetts Institute of Technology (MIT), Cambridge, Mass. Their classic paper, *"The Hallmarks of Cancer,"* was published in *Cell* in 2000 and revised and expanded as "the Next Generation" in 2011.

"Hallmarks" is the most cited paper in *Cell's* history, having been referenced more than 27,550 times! Weinberg amplified the paper's central message in a 796-page textbook, *The Biology of Cancer (2007)*. These two papers, Weinberg's massive book, and a summary chapter in the world's most influential cancer textbook, have become the organizational framework for almost everyone seriously engaged in understanding cancer. This fundamental orientation has increasingly been incorporated into the thinking of most CAM-oriented physicians and scientists as well.
(D. Hanahan, R.A. Weinberg. The hallmarks of cancer. *Cell,* 100 (2000), pp. 57–70; Hanahan, Douglas, and Robert A. Weinberg. *"Hallmarks of Cancer: The next Generation."* Cell 144, no. 5 (March 4, 2011): 646–74; Weinberg, Robert A. The Biology of Cancer, New York: Garland Science, 2007)

We, therefore, need to understand the fundamental features of cancer, and then devise practical plans based on that knowledge. We also need to focus on those aspects of the problem that the patient can influence. The word patient itself is problematic, since it implies passivity. Its first meaning (dating from the early 14th century) was "bearing pains or trials calmly or without complaint." Only later was this applied to the recipient of medical care.

Patients cannot do much about their genetic inheritance but they can often control their immediate environment, including food and drink, exercise and activity, supplement usage, and to a degree, mental and emotional outlook.

Background

In 2000, the two distinguished scientists, Drs. Douglas Hanahan and Robert A. Weinberg published their summary of the six major "Hallmarks of Cancer".

These hallmarks included the following:

- Sustaining proliferative signaling
- Evading growth suppressors
- Resisting cell death
- Enabling replicative immortality
- Inducing angiogenesis
- Activating invasion and metastasis

In 2011, Hanahan and Weinberg updated this list as "The Hallmarks of Cancer: The Next Generation." Under the influence or prodding of CAM-friendly scientists (such as James D. Watson, Ph.D.) they added four "new" causative factors:

- Genomic instability
- Reprogramming of energy metabolism
- Evading immune destruction
- The tumor microenvironment

Although they stated at the time that they were adding these factors "because of conceptual progress in the last decade," it happens that these four are among the oldest theories of cancer. Genomic instability was the theory of Theodor Boveri, MD (1862-1915); energy metabolism was part of the astonishing life work of Otto H. Warburg, MD, Ph.D. (1883-1970); evading immune destruction is a concept that dates back to Paul Ehrlich, MD Ph.D. (1854-1915); and "the tumor microenvironment" dates to the work of Stephen Paget, MD (1855-1926).

As you can see, all of these "new" advances actually date from the late 19th and early 20th centuries! In fact, what is astonishing is that Hanahan and Weinberg could have missed these in their first iteration of the hallmarks. But better late than never. Or, to quote Scripture:

"What has been will be again, what has been done will be done again; there is nothing new under the sun" (Ecclesiastes 1:9)

Nonetheless, these two publications have had a profound impact on the way the scientific world thinks about the cancer problem. However, to our way of thinking, they failed to prioritize these hallmarks, or to pull them all into a credible theory of cancer. For example, they only glancingly referred to fundamental facts about cancer that individuals can influence. To us, these three things are profoundly true, scientifically documented, and actionable by the patient, with or even without the help of holistic practitioners.

Hanahan and Weinberg allude to these three, especially in their 2011 revision. We always keep these three principles in mind. Yet these are rarely ever mentioned, much less explained, to the average cancer patient. Here they are:

1. Cancer has a faulty metabolism.

As Prof. Thomas N. Seyfried of Boston College has said, cancer is a metabolic disease. This is what Hanahan and Weinberg call "reprogramming of energy metabolism." So what exactly is "energy metabolism"? The National Cancer Institute dictionary defines metabolism as follows:

"The chemical changes that take place in a cell or an organism. These changes make energy, and the materials cells and organisms need to grow, reproduce and stay healthy. Metabolism also helps get rid of toxic substances."

For instance, it is readily observable that cancer cells typically produce lactate (lactic acid). This has been known since Warburg's great discovery of 1924. But why is this? It was Warburg's theory that cancer cells have lost most of their ability to generate energy efficiently through normal respiration (a process scientists call oxidative phosphorylation, abbreviated OxPhos.)

That, in turn, occurred because cancer cells have lost a complete or fully functioning set of mitochondria, where any mammalian cell's energy is normally generated. To elude death, these defective cells then revert to a primitive form of energy generation, called aerobic glycolysis. The result is a cell that is avid for glucose (the form that carbohydrates normally take in the blood). Cancer cells crave and devour glucose because they must primarily use it in this intrinsically inefficient way.

This one fact presents several powerful treatment opportunities, such as "mito-oncology" proposed by Nobel laureate James D. Watson, and colleagues.

2. A properly functioning immune system protects against cancer.

This is what Hanahan and Weinberg refer to as cancer cells "evading immune destruction". Immune cells (mainly lymphocytes classified as "T" and "NK" cells) represent the body's innate defense against cancer. Lymphocytes are involved in every phase of the cancer process, although sometimes they may be subverted by cancer itself. However, the effectiveness of the immune response to cancer can be enhanced by immune modulators and checkpoint inhibitors. External factors, such as medicinal mushrooms, certain herbs such as astragalus, and food factors such as curcumin and sulforaphane, can influence the immune response. Instead, most chemotherapy has a negative effect on the immune system (plummeting lymphocytes, neutrophils and other types of white blood cells), which completely contradicts the goal of fostering the immune system to destroy the tumor.

3. The root cause of this disease is a cancer stem cell (CSC).

All cells in a tumor are not created equal. There is a hierarchy within tumors, with cancer stem cells (CSCs) at the peak of the pyramid. These stem cells are many, many times more malignant than the usual cancer cell. Many scientists believe that CSCs create and organize the entire tumor. Cancer's growth, recurrence, and metastases are driven by the activity of CSCs.

For Hanahan and Weinberg, cancer stem cells do not (yet) rise to the level of a key hallmark of cancer. Here is what they say:

"Although the evidence is still fragmentary, CSCs may prove to be a common constituent of many if not most tumors, albeit being present with widely varying abundance. CSCs are defined operationally through their ability to efficiently seed new tumors upon inoculation into recipient host mice (Cho and Clarke, 2008, Lobo et al., 2007). This functional definition is often complemented by including the expression in CSCs of markers that are also expressed by the normal stem cells in the tissue-of-origin (Al-Hajj et al., 2003)."

The cancer stem cell (CSC) has its origin in the work of the great pathologists of the late 19th and early 20th centuries: Robert Remak, MD (1815-1865), the inventor of the theory that all cells come from pre-existing cells; Rudolph Virchow, MD (1821-1902); his star pupil, Julius F. Cohnheim, MD (1839-1884) and John Beard, Ph.D. of Edinburgh (1858-1924).

It is odd that Hanahan and Weinberg consider the evidence for CSC to be "still fragmentary," but perhaps that was the case in 2011, when they published the "Next Generation" article. Their comments on CSCs, while highly technical, are worthwhile. And their ultimate conclusions are positive:

"These complexities notwithstanding, it is evident that this new dimension of tumor heterogeneity holds important implications for successful cancer therapies. Increasing evidence in a variety of tumor types suggests that cells with properties of CSCs are more resistant to various commonly used chemotherapeutic treatments." (Singh and Settleman, 2010, Creighton et al., 2009, Buck et al., 2007).

"Their persistence may help to explain the almost-inevitable disease recurrence following apparently successful debulking of human solid tumors by radiation and various forms of chemotherapy". Indeed, CSCs may well prove to underlie certain forms of tumor dormancy, whereby latent cancer cells persist for years or even decades after surgical resection or radio/chemotherapy, only to suddenly erupt and generate life-threatening disease.

Hence, CSCs may represent a double-threat, in that they are more resistant to therapeutic killing and, at the same time, endowed with the ability to regenerate a tumor once therapy has been halted."

This is the most cogent explanation we have of all the worst activities of cancer (drug resistance, recurrences, and metastases). In their next revision, if there is to be one, Hanahan and Weinberg should not only put the CSC theory among the "hallmarks," but they should put it at the top of their list, because it does so much to explain so many other subsidiary aspects of the disease.

Much remains to be understood about CSCs, of course, and there are key points of debate (which, in our opinion, has kept the Nobel Prize committee from recognizing John Dick, Ph.D., (Toronto), Max Wicha, MD (Michigan), Michael F. Clarke, M.D. (Stanford) or other pioneers of this important concept.

This didn't stop the Nobel Prize committee from recognizing James P. Allison, Ph.D, and Tasuku Honjo, MD, Ph.D, in 2018. We would suggest that the big difference is that the work on immunotherapy had already resulted in several blockbuster drugs (ipilimumab, nivolumab, pembrolizumab, etc.) whereas the work of CSCs has been unable to come up with a single practical drug.

Nonetheless, the work on cancer stem cells continues apace, and is slowly gaining adherents in the conservative field of oncology. There are at this writing over 18,000 PubMed-indexed articles on the concept. New ones are appearing at a rate of almost 2,000 per year. The CSC concept has been demonstrated in all the major cancer types.

THE NEUTROPHIL-TO-LYMPHOCYTE RATIO (NLR) AND WHY IT'S IMPORTANT

How can you tell if your immune system is deficient? One simple way to tell if your immune system is deficient is to learn how to interpret your complete blood count (CBC). If any of the numbers are too high or too low (indicated by the letter "H" or "L" next to the score) this is a clear indication of a problem.

But there is a quick and efficient way that (although well known to physicians) patients are rarely told about. Doctors either ignore this or don't feel their patients need to know it. This is a calculation of your physiological stress level. It is called the **NLR**, which stands for the **"neutrophil-to-lymphocyte ratio."**

The NLR is of particular importance to cancer patients. The importance of this ratio was first described in 1967 as a way to measure exposure to toxic ozone gas. Its relevance to cancer was initiated in 2014 by a study in the Journal of the National Cancer Institute (JNCI), which surveyed 100 journal articles that included a total of 40,559 cancer patients. The authors concluded that an NLR **greater than four** was associated with **an 81% increase** in death. This was observed in all types of cancer, all sites, and all stages.

The NLR is an **open secret**. There are about 100 new papers on the topic every month. It is, in short, "an easily accessible prognostic marker." Yet, we have not met a patient aware of this fact.

Since the NLR measures both inflammation and immunity, it serves as an early warning system for death of all kinds. Another study found that this simple and inexpensive test was remarkably accurate in predicting an impending catastrophe:

"The NLR is a predictor of all-cause mortality and cardiovascular events" (edited).

Simply put, people who score high on the NLR also have about double the risk of dying of heart attacks, strokes, or any cause compared to people with low-normal NLR scores.

Why is this number so critical? The NLR measures the relationship between two key blood components. It is beneficial to have a high normal number of lymphocytes, 1,800 (1.8K) or higher, because lymphocytes include the most active cancer-killing cells. In other words, from the point of view of cancer, lymphocytes are critically important. On the other hand, neutrophils are associated with chronic inflammation, which can be the seedbed of tumors:

*"**Neutrophils reflect a state of host inflammation, which is a hallmark of cancer.** They can participate in different stages of the cancer process including tumor initiation, growth, proliferation, or metastatic spread. In general, neutrophils play a central role in inflammation within the tumor."*
(Ocana A, Nieto-Jiménez C, Pandiella A, Templeton AJ. Neutrophils in cancer: prognostic role and therapeutic strategies. Mol Cancer. 2017;16(1):137. Published 2017 Aug 15. doi:10.1186/s12943-017-0707-7, edited)

A dozen authorities from five countries concluded:

"A high NLR [of over 4.0] is associated with an adverse overall survival in many solid tumors. The NLR is a readily available and inexpensive biomarker."

Since few patients know about it, you might think this discovery is obscure. Not at all. It has had over 10,000 views, and 5,000+ downloads, and has been cited by 800+ other publications!

To emphasize this point, here is how the NLR correlates with a worse prognosis in some cancer situations:

Lung Cancer (NSCLC):

"Elevated pretreatment NLR is associated with shorter overall survival and progression-free survival and with lower response rates in patients with metastatic lung cancer (NSCLC) treated with nivolumab immunotherapy, independently of other prognostic factors."
(Diem S, Schmid S, Krapf M, et al. Neutrophil-to-Lymphocyte ratio (NLR) and Platelet-to-Lymphocyte ratio (PLR) as prognostic markers in patients with non-small cell lung cancer (NSCLC) treated with nivolumab. Lung Cancer. 2017 Sep;111:176-181. doi: 10.1016/j.

lungcan.2017.07.024. Epub 2017 Jul 24. PMID: 28838390, edited)

Breast Cancer (triple-negative breast cancer):

High NLR is associated with poor **overall survival** and disease-free survival in patients with breast cancer, especially in those patients with estrogen receptor (ER-) and HER2-negative disease." There is no mention of the progesterone receptor (PR) status, but this finding might be relevant to those with triple-negative disease.

Stomach Cancer (gastric adenocarcinoma):

In the high-NLR patients, there was a four times greater chance of postoperative complications. The median survival time was 216 days shorter in the high-NLR patient group and disease-free survival was approximately half.
(Miyamoto R, Inagawa S, Sano N, et al. The neutrophil-to-lymphocyte ratio (NLR) predicts short-term and long-term outcomes in gastric cancer patients. Eur J Surg Oncol. 2018 May;44(5):607-612. doi: 10.1016/j.ejso.2018.02.003. Epub 2018 Feb 13. PMID: 29478743)

Melanoma:

"NLR is a simple, inexpensive, and readily available biomarker that could be used to help predict response to immunotherapy in patients with advanced melanoma."

There are similar findings on almost every major kind of cancer, including esophagus, liver, cervix, ovarian, colorectal, and head-and-neck cancer.

How to Calculate Your NLR

You can calculate your NLR by dividing the number of neutrophils by the number of lymphocytes from a typical CBC blood test. (You can also divide the *percentage* of neutrophils by the *percentage* of lymphocytes, and the results will be the same. But you cannot compare one absolute number to one *percentage* number.)

The Neutrophil-Lymphocyte Ratio (NLR) Calculator app (type in *MDCalc Medical Calculator* in the APP Store to download) allows you to enter either the absolute numbers or the percentage of these two WBCs to perform the calculation. [But please don't mix and match absolute numbers and percentages.] Again, if we enter an absolute number of 3.0 for the neutrophils and **1.5** for the lymphocytes, the actual number is **1.5**. But the calculator will simply round off to the number TWO. This indicates normal physiological stress, but it isn't very exact.

If you can't find the absolute numbers, you can usually find the percentages. Thus, if the percent of neutrophils is **53.6%**, while lymphocytes is **33.2%**, **it will again return** a score of TWO, which is NORMAL.

What is a Normal NLR Score?

There is general agreement that a high NLR score is associated with an increased risk of disease and death. But there is no universal agreement on what constitutes a normal score. We have seen estimates ranging from 2.5 to 4.0, or even higher. But the most convincing study came from Patrice Forget, MD, clinical professor of anesthesiology at the University of Aberdeen. In the study, routine blood samples were obtained from 413 healthy individuals, who had a median age of 38. This study established that the normal NLR values in an adult, non-geriatric, population in good health were between **0.78 and 3.53**. The average (mean) number was **1.65**.

This tells us that the normal NLR number is likely to be between 1 and 3, with 1.65 as probably ideal. The normal NLR value in an adult, non-geriatric population in good health is between 0.78 and 3.53. So an NLR higher than 3.53 suggests stress, inflammation, or infection in your body.

Here is how to calculate the NLR based on a standard Complete Blood Count (CBC):

Locate the absolute neutrophil number. (This may be abbreviated as ABS. NEUTS or some such designation.) Let's say, by way of example, that this number is **3.0**.

Next, find the absolute lymphocyte number. (This may be abbreviated as ABS. LYMPHS.) Let's say this number is **1.5**.

Divide the number of neutrophils (3.0) by the number of lymphocytes (1.5). This will yield an NLR of 1.5. Since anything below the cut-off point of 3.53 is average for healthy young adults, 1.5 represents a normal score.

ALKALINE PHOSPHATASE	1054 H	35-144 U/L
AST	24	10-35 U/L
ALT	5 L	9-46 U/L
DIFFERENTIAL, MANUAL		
→ ABSOLUTE NEUTROPHILS	2597	1500-7800 cells/uL
ABSOLUTE BAND NEUTROPHILS	294	0-750 cells/uL
→ ABSOLUTE LYMPHOCYTES	1519	850-3900 cells/uL
ABSOLUTE MONOCYTES	343	200-950 cells/uL
[illegible]	[illegible]	[illegible]

In the above example, the two black arrows represent the absolute neutrophils (2597) and the absolute lymphocytes (1519). The ratio is **1.7**, which is normal.

You can also use the online NLR calculator.

What to do about a high Neutrophil-Lymphocyte Ratio (NLR)?

Some cancer patients have abnormally high NLRs (which, as a reminder, Prof. Forget defines as over 3.53). This could represent either one problem, or two problems converging in the same individual. In other words, these patients may have a low number of lymphocytes (often due to the effects of toxic treatments) or it can be due to an unusually high number of neutrophils. This is usually due to some inflammatory condition. Or both, simultaneously.

But what can you do about either, or both, of these problems?

Treatments that reduce systemic inflammation and/or enhance anticancer immunity are intended to raise the too-low numbers of lymphocytes, or reduce too-high numbers of neutrophils, thereby rebalancing the neutrophil to lymphocyte ratio.

Much of our effort is directed at optimizing these two underlying situations (decreasing chronic inflammation and increasing immune potency).

There is good evidence that medicinal mushrooms and **traditional Asian medicine (TCM, Ayurveda, Kampo, etc.)** will lower the neutrophil-to-lymphocyte ratio. In 2013, Japanese scientists looked at changes in the NLR in patients who had previously undergone surgery for colorectal cancer. Patients were classified into those with a higher NLR versus a lower NLR.

(Their cut-off point was 2.5, which was more rigorous than the 3.53 cited above.)

Each patient was given chemotherapy plus a registered anticancer medicine called PSK (polysaccharide K)) derived from shiitake mushrooms. In patients who began the trial with a relatively high NLR, "the use of postoperative **PSK-chemotherapy controlled the NLR at low levels**." But patients who began the trial with a low NLR "tended to remain low." The authors concluded:

"In patients who underwent colorectal cancer surgery, postoperative adjuvant therapy with a combination of chemotherapy and PSK [medicinal mushrooms] succeeded in controlling the NLR at low levels."
(Yoshioka S, Kubo M, Yanagisawa K, et al. [Clinical significance of neutrophil to lymphocyte ratio in colorectal cancer patients receiving adjuvant chemotherapy combined with polysaccharide-K]. Gan To Kagaku Ryoho. 2013 Nov;40(12):2086-8. Japanese. PMID: 24394021)

This is a very important statement. It confirms our belief that good mushroom extracts should be efficacious in this situation.

As to lowering chronic inflammation, one can take nonsteroidal anti-inflammatory drugs (NSAIDs), such as ibuprofen. You can read about these at the always helpful website, drugs.com. NSAIDs come with risks of their own, especially with long-term use. There is evidence, however, that some of the nutraceuticals (dietary supplements that are believed to provide health benefits) are quite effective at reducing inflammation. For a full list of recommended nutraceuticals, see www.themossreport.com.

MOLECULAR AND GENOMIC TESTING

This is among the most important topics in oncology. Since this report is written for lay *people, I will focus on the primary question: whether or not live, frozen or preserved tissue can be analyzed at the molecular level to yield actionable information on treatment?* Clearly, in some cases, it can.

Background: The earliest molecular test was for estrogen receptors (ER+) in breast tumors. If a patient's tumor proved positive for estrogen receptors, it was recommended that she be given the drug tamoxifen to counteract that receptor. Depending on the patient, taking this oral drug every day might add as much as a ten-percentage-point increase in the chances of survival at ten or fifteen years.
((http://www.predict.nhs.uk/predict.html; Tamoxifen dates from 1960 although it only came into widespread use in the 1970s. Kistner, R. W., and O. W. Smith. Observations on the Use of a Non-Steroidal Estrogen Antagonist: MER-25. Surgical Forum 1960:10:725–29.

The discovery by Watson and Crick of the double helix structure of DNA in 1953, and then the sequencing of the 19,000 to 20,000 protein coding genes in the human genome, has led to an explosion of knowledge about the molecular and genetic nature of many things, including cancer. The cost of DNA analysis has fallen precipitously, but the number of cancer markers has risen.

Cancer genome sequencing has focused on the "SNPs," or single nucleotide polymorph sms. A SNP (pronounced "snip") is a variation in a single base pair in a DNA sequence. Identifying such mutations is increasingly common in laboratories around the world. These tests are fairly routine now for breast cancer, various kinds of leukemia and lymphoma, some forms of lung cancer, and other tumors as well. "Companion tests" are frequently approved along with new drugs. **Everyone** with a particular type of cancer is a candidate for the test, while those who are positive for the mutation in question also get the very expensive companion drug.

There are also a number of laboratories that offer companion testing directly to patients or to complementary doctors.

While normal whole genome sequencing is based on blood cells, saliva, etc., when it comes to cancer, scientists analyze tissue, either from the primary tumor, from metastatic lesions or occasionally from a blood sample. The information that comes from this process is the identification of DNA or RNA, or the number of copies, mutations, translocations or fusions of genes. All of these abnormalities are characteristic of cancer. They correspond to Hanahan and Weinberg's **cancer hallmark, unstable DNA**, with its various strange combinations, deletions, and movement or "translocation" of genes.

There are mutations of various kinds in cancers, but most of the drugs approved by the U.S. Food and Drug Administration (FDA) in the past 20 or so years have, in one way or another, targeted these mutations or other abnormal qualities of the cancer, such as new blood vessel formation (angiogenesis).

Oncology has evolved towards the incorporation of targeted agents in many treatment protocols. This is almost always done in combination with cytotoxic chemotherapy. In some cases, though, genomic testing is not done to determine treatment. Instead, treatment protocols are administered as per predetermined protocols.

There are some built-in limitations to targeted drugs. These include the following:

- Cancers, as they evolve, are prone to multiple mutations. If you suppress one mutation, the cancer may find other abnormal growth pathways.
- Many genetic abnormalities do not have corresponding drugs.
- The existing drugs attack non-critical mutations but not the crucial "driver mutations" of the tumor.
- Targeted drugs may cause serious side effects, especially when used in combination. This limits one's ability to create combinations that might cover the majority of mutations.

For more information and Dr. Moss' insights on targeted drugs and a plausible solution to these limitations, visit www.themossreport.com.

CANCERS OF UNKNOWN PRIMARY SITE (CUPS)

One useful test is CancerTYPE ID, from Biotheranostics, Inc. This is a 92-gene expression assay, which classifies tumors by matching the gene expression pattern of a patient's cancer cells to a database of 50 known tumor types, covering more than 95 percent of all solid tumors. The assay analyzes tissue-specific tumor markers to distinguish between the various tumor types and subtypes. Since its launch in 2008, more than 7,500 oncologists and more than 5,000 pathologists have used CancerTYPE ID. The test results are available five days after receipt of the sample and the required information. It is completely covered by Medicare.

The CancerTYPE ID test provides "actionable genomic information for accurate diagnosis for metastatic patients with diagnostic ambiguity." This is the best test I know of to pinpoint the type of cancer that a person is dealing with.

THE TNM CANCER STAGING SYSTEM

The TNM system is an almost universally adopted method of classifying all solid tumors by reference to three key characteristics. These are the size and extent of the tumors (the "T" in TNM), the spread of cancer to the lymph nodes (the "N"), and the extent of nonlocal metastases (the "M"). Two organizations, the American Joint Committee on Cancer (AJCC) and the Union for International Cancer Control (UICC), maintain the TNM classification system worldwide to help doctors determine the stage of many different types of cancer, based on common standards.

In the TNM system, the stage is determined AFTER cancer has been assigned a letter or number to describe the key features of this particular disease. The TNM score briefly summarizes crucial information that helps assign this particular cancer to its current **stage**. This is a process of determining the degree to which any particular cancer has grown or spread. Typically, doctors assign a Roman numeral from I to IV to any solid cancer. The letter "I" refers to an isolated tumor, while IV is cancer that has spread distantly (or is at its greatest extent).

Here is a more detailed description of the various TNM categories. We have borrowed it from the ACS website:

The Primary Tumor (T category)

The **T category** can be assigned a letter or a number:

- **TX** means there's no information about the primary tumor, or it can't be measured.
- **T0** means there is no evidence of a primary tumor (it cannot be found).
- **Tis** means that the cancer cells are only growing in the layer of cells where they started, without growing into deeper layers. This may also be called **in situ** cancer or **pre-cancer**.

A number after the T (such as **T1, T2, T3, or T4**) might describe the tumor size and/or amount of spread into nearby structures. The higher the T number, the larger the tumor and/or the more it has grown into nearby tissues.

The Lymph Nodes (N category)

Lymph nodes near the primary tumor are usually checked to find out if cancer has spread into them. Lymph nodes are small, bean-shaped collections of immune cells. Many types of cancer often spread to nearby lymph nodes before they reach other parts of the body.

- The **N** category can be assigned a letter or a number:
- **NX** means there's no information about the nearby lymph nodes, or they can't be assessed.
- **N0** means nearby lymph nodes do not contain cancer.
- A number after the **N** (such as **N1, N2, or N3)** might describe the size, location, and/or the number of nearby lymph nodes affected by cancer. The higher the N number, the more cancer has spread to nearby lymph nodes.

Cancer Metastasis (M category)

Doctors might also look at other parts of the body to see if cancer has spread. Cancer that has spread to parts of the body far from the primary tumor is known as **metastasis** and contributes to the staging equation.

The **M category** is assigned a number:

- **M0** means that no distant cancer spread has been found.
- **M1** means that cancer has been found to have spread to distant organs or tissues.

Typically, doctors use the TNM system when talking among themselves. The end result of this is to assign a **stage** to cancer. Patients are usually only made aware of the stage of their cancer, not their TNM status, which is a more technical item.

Correlating Cancer Staging Systems

A question we are frequently asked is, *"How does one correlate these two systems?"* In other words, a person might know their stage but not their actual TNM ranking, or vice versa.

It might seem like a straightforward question but it is anything but. The topic is complicated because other factors can influence the determination of the stage. And particular cancers may have their own separate staging system. But as a general rule, to quote the NCI website, most staging systems will include information about:

- Where the tumor is located in the body
- The cell type (such as adenocarcinoma or squamous cell carcinoma)
- The size of the tumor
- Whether cancer has spread to nearby lymph nodes
- Whether cancer has spread to a different part of the body

Tumor grade refers to how abnormal the cancer cells look and how likely the tumor is to grow

TABLE 45.2

2017 American Joint Committee on Cancer Overall Stage Grouping

When T Is ...	And N Is ...	And M Is ...	Then the Stage Group Is ...
T1	N0	M0	I
T2	N0	M0	II
T3	N0	M0	III
T1, T2, T3	N1	M0	III
T4a	N0, N1	M0	IVA
T1, T2, T3, T4a	N2	M0	IVAt
Any T	N3	M0	IVB
T4b	Any N	M0	IVB
Any T	Any N	M1	IVC

Used with the permission of the American College of Surgeons. The original source for this material is the AJCC Cancer Staging Manual, Eighth Edition (2017) published by Springer International Publishing AG.

Thus, in this particular case, only small tumors with no lymph node involvement and no distant metastasis constitute stage I cancer. A larger primary tumor but still with no lymph nodes or distant metastases is stage II cancer. A still larger tumor with no lymph node or distant metastasis is stage III cancer. But ANY size tumor with lymph node involvement is also stage III. And a very large tumor with any or 1 lymph node involvement is considered stage IV cancer, as is extensive lymph node involvement. ANY degree of distant metastasis with or without any primary tumor or any lymph node involvement is automatically a "stage IVC" tumor, which is the highest stage possible.

But bear in mind that there are over 100 types of cancer, and the staging system for each of them may vary from case to case. Anyone needing further detailed information on this topic should definitely acquire the following classic text:

AJCC Cancer Staging Manual, Eighth Edition

TREATMENT

SURGERY

In general, *The Moss Report* does not get into long or involved discussions of the techniques of surgery for any type of cancer. I agree that surgery is often an indispensable and foundational treatment for cancer. But the discussion of surgical technique is far too technical for the non-specialist reader. Questions of surgical technique for various kinds of cancer are rooted deep in the past. They evolved from a time when surgery was a trade, which followed the apprenticeship model that was characteristic of other trades. Even with the present-day's rigorous scientific education, "many traditional components and philosophies of surgical training continue to apply today." As a result, statistics regarding the outcome of various surgical techniques are often not as formalized as they are for more modern treatments, such as chemotherapy. (Polavarpu, Harsha V., Afif N. Kulaylat, Susie Sun, and Osama H. Hamed. "100 Years of Surgical Education: The Past, Present, and Future." Bulletin of the American College of Surgeons 98, no 7 (July 2013):22-27)

While I may address innovative surgery techniques, wherever appropriate, I confess to a strong preference for so-called "conservative surgery," i.e., removing as little tissue as possible, within the bounds of safety. My philosophy was shaped by the rise of the partial mastectomy or lumpectomy in the 1970s. Conservative surgery was first advocated by a British surgeon who performed a partial nephrectomy for kidney cancer in 1899. He wrote:

"The tendency of all the operations of modern surgery is towards conservation, whenever permissible and legitimate."
(Moynihan, B. G. Partial nephrectomy. British Medical Journal 1, no. 2144 (February 1, 1902): 263–65)

That saying should have been engraved over the doorway of every surgical theater in the world! But the era of radical surgery was just dawning, and lasted well into the 1980s. In fact, it isn't entirely over yet. Each case has to be examined on its own merits, but as a general rule the less cutting, the better.

RADIATION

According to the National Cancer Institute, about half of all cancer patients receive radiation as a part of their treatment. Ionizing radiation, such as radium and X-rays, has been a part of cancer treatment since the days of the Nobel laureate **Madame Marie Curie** (1867-1934) in the 1920s and 1930s. Some techniques now involve huge and costly machinery. Proton beam accelerators can cost $150 million!

In essence, radiation comes down to finding more efficient ways of focusing a destructive beam with great accuracy on a tumor while inflicting less damage on surrounding healthy tissues. (Chetty, et al 2015)

Like most things in science, claims of effectiveness should be subjected to rigorous experimental tests. This is sometimes lacking with radiation studies. At this writing, there is no rigorous evidence that proton beam therapy is better than the older photon-based radiation treatments. Nonetheless, taken together, the newer technique seems like a significant refinement of this century-old modality. At the very least, today's radiation treatment is less of an ordeal than the version that our grandparents suffered through decades ago. (Mould, 1995)

However, the number of peer-reviewed articles on the topic of radiation therapy for cancer stood at approximately 300,000, including 20,000 or so clinical trial citations, providing a vast library of research on the topic. We cannot hope to do more than skim the surface in this guide.

Instead, I will focus on those techniques that show the greatest promise. Because techniques change, evolve and improve so quickly, radiotherapy is constantly reinventing itself. (http://www.cancer.gov/cancertopics/factsheet/therapy/radiation)

There are several relatively new or unusual forms of radiation therapy (or radiotherapy, as it is more formally called). Most of these are better ways of focusing a beam of radiation so that it targets the tumor with greater accuracy and inflicts less damage on surrounding normal tissues. (Calabrese P, et al, 2009)

The "new radiotherapy" is sometimes used in conjunction with other treatments, in an attempt to minimize toxicity and/or increase effectiveness as well.

Despite much hype, no form of radiation treatment is entirely without risk. Nor is it well established through randomized clinical trials (RCTs) that some of these techniques extend the overall survival of the patients who are treated. One often hears the claim that clinical results with radiation are bound to improve because of their increasing ability to target tumors more accurately and spare normal tissue. This hypothesis needs to be rigorously tested.

Innovative Forms of Radiation: Broadly Categorized

Restricted (or limited) Field Techniques

These are techniques in which the beam is tightly focused on the cancerous target. This is currently one of the most active areas of investigation in the field of radiation (over 2,000 PubMed citations). Often when oncologists speak of the 'cutting edge' of radiation therapy, they are referring to the use of one of the following four restricted field techniques.

- Conformal Radiation Therapy (CRT)
- Intraoperative Radiation Therapy (IORT)
- Gamma Knife® Surgery and
- Stereotactic Radiation Therapy.

(Yamashita H, Okuma K, Wakui R, et al. Details of recurrence sites after elective nodal irradiation (ENI) using 3D-conformal radiotherapy (3D-CRT) combined with chemotherapy for thoracic esophageal squamous cell carcinoma - A retrospective analysis. Radiother Oncol. 2010. Available at: http://www.ncbi.nlm.nih.gov/pubmed/21074880)

Extended Field Techniques

An alternative strategy is to use an extended field in order to encompass more of the body in the X-rays, thereby denying the tumor a safe haven from which to grow back. These techniques include:

- Total Body Irradiation (TBI)
- Radioimmunotherapy (radiolabeled antibodies such as Zevalin and Bexxar)

Stratification Techniques

Another approach is to modify the timing of delivering radiation, a technique known as stratification or fractionation:

- Modified fractionation schemes
- CHART (continuous hyperfractionated accelerated radiation therapy) particularly used

in the treatment of non-small cell lung cancer.

Body Radiosurgery

Body Radiosurgery is commonly used in the treatment of brain tumors. But it can, ideally, be used in the treatment of non-cranial sites as well. In the U.S., the most prominent advocate and practitioner of fractionated stereotactic radiation therapy for non-cranial sites has been Gilbert S. Lederman, MD (www.rsny.org).

According to Lederman, “The success rate (control of the cancer in the treated site) is high and the durability of treatment is usually for the remainder of the patient’s life.” Notice the wording. This does not mean that the patient necessarily has a prolongation of life span—only that the sites that are irradiated do not become cancerous again.

I believe that the introduction of body radiosurgery has been a positive development, offering increased choices to cancer patients. However, there is a surprising lack of randomized controlled trials (RCTs) to support the claims of this cancer treatment.

Modified Fractionation Schemes

These are innovative schedules that adjust the time frame in which radiation is delivered. This is done in order to decrease the toxicity of treatment and increase the total amount of radiation that can be delivered to the tumor. The most common modifications involve hyperfractionation, which means dividing the conventional amount of radiation into two or three treatment sessions per day.

The rationale for *hyperfractionation* is that since human cancer cells can proliferate rapidly, dividing the dose of radiation therapy into more frequent sessions may more effectively eradicate tumor cells while simultaneously reducing the long-term damage to normal tissues.

Extended Field Therapies

As the names imply, extended field therapies start from the opposite philosophy of limited (or restricted) field therapy. The goal of this group of therapies is to *increase* the area of the body exposed to radiation. This group of treatments includes lymphatic, half body and total body irradiation (TBI), as well as targeted radionuclides, which are radioactive drugs administered systemically.

Radiation Sensitizers and Protectors

Various substances, including drugs and nutritional supplements, can be used to modify the effects of radiation. Substances called *radiosensitizers* (efaproxiral, for example) can make cancer cells more susceptible to the damaging effects of ionizing rays. Many chemotherapy agents also do that, which partially accounts for the enhanced effect of using combined modality treatments (also known as chemoradiation).
(Mohindra P, Sinha RN, Andrews RJ, Khuntia D. Non-cytotoxic radiosensitizers in brain radiotherapy: journey till the first decade of this millennium. Curr Cancer Drug Targets. 2012;12(3):260–278)

There are also substances that help spare normal tissues from radiation’s damage. The FDA has approved three such agents as radioprotectors. These are *Amifostine, Mesna* and *ICRF-187.* They are all synthetic antioxidants, created in chemistry labs to mimic (and presumably improve upon) the effects of dietary antioxidants. These agents are sometimes used by oncologists to lessen the severity of radiation and chemotherapy. For instance, use of the toxic drug ifosfamide would be virtually impossible without Mesna, which protects against otherwise unacceptable damage to the bladder.

All three of these drugs have been extensively investigated in the laboratory and clinic, and all have been found to be relatively safe and effective. The use of these synthetic antioxidants is not a subject of controversy, and oncologists, as a rule, no longer worry that they will interfere with radiation or chemotherapy. In fact, doctors use them precisely in order to reduce the side effects of conventional treatment. But synthetic antioxidants may have side effects of their own.

Their use raises the interesting question of whether nutritional supplements, which are generally available over the counter, and are as a rule better tolerated than synthetic drugs, could be used in similar protective ways. This question often elicits vigorous debate and even outright hostility from some oncologists. The question of whether one should take antioxidants during conventional cancer therapy is one that continues to cause great controversy among researchers, patients and physicians.

CT or MRI?

At some point, your doctor may offer you a choice of having a computed tomography (CT or CAT) or a magnetic resonance imaging (MRI) scan. Always choose the MRI. There is a big difference between the two in radiation exposure, because an MRI involves no ionizing radiation, but relies on giant magnets to get a detailed look inside the body. A CT scan is a kind of motion picture X-ray, which exposes you to considerable ionizing radiation. This is ironic because radiation itself is a known cause of cancer. So choose not to take a test that can sometimes cause cancer in order to find out if you have cancer!

According to an excellent report from Consumer Reports:

"CT emits a powerful dose of radiation, in some cases equivalent to about 200 chest X- rays, or the amount most people would be exposed to from natural sources over seven years. That dose can alter the makeup of human tissue and create free radicals, molecules that can wreak havoc on human cells. Your body can often repair that damage—but not always. And when it doesn't, the damage can lead to cancer." (http://www.consumerreports.org/cro/magazine/2015/01/the-surprising-dangers-of-ct-sans-and-x-rays/index.htm)

The same holds true for other cancers as well. Consumer Reports states that about 15,000 people die every year because of cancers that are caused by the radiation in CT scans alone. But, in a survey of over 1,000 U.S. adults, they found that people are seldom told by their doctors about the risks of CT scans or other radiological tests. Only seven percent of those who had a non-dental X-ray and only two percent of those who had a CT scan thought they might have received the tests unnecessarily. And just four percent told their doctor they did not want a CT scan. The neurologist Orly Avitzur, MD, of Tarrytown, NY, said:

"That's worrisome. Patients need to take the lead on this because their doctor may not."

There are times when your doctors may insist on a CT scan. That is because CTs sometimes do things that MRIs cannot do. They can outline bones inside the body very accurately. Also, a CT of the brain is much faster to arrange than an MRI. In such cases, it makes perfect sense to accept the risks of radiation for the benefit of quickly assessing medical conditions.

CHEMOTHERAPY

"Do not neglect medical treatment when it is necessary, but leave it off when health has been

restored. Treat disease through diet, by preference, refraining from the use of drugs. Abstain from drugs when the health is good, but administer them when necessary."

—Bahá'u'lláh (1817-1892), Tablet to a Physician (http://bahai-library.com/uhj_lawh_tibb)

Chemotherapy has been much criticized for its obvious deficiencies. It causes many serious side effects, not all of which can be overcome by other treatments. Despite what the patient goes through, cancer all too often finds a way around "chemo," and can recur or persist despite it. These are the harsh realities for many patients. But although one may be philosophically opposed to the introduction of poisons into an already sick body, the truth is that many lives have been extended, and some people have even been cured, through the use of this radical type of intervention. Sometimes the immediate effects of chemotherapy are truly remarkable!

There is no need to repeat here all of the arguments regarding the use of chemotherapy. More than 25 years ago, I wrote a book on the topic, *Questioning Chemotherapy*, and followed it up with another book on the general topic, *Customized Cancer Treatment.*

It would be unbalanced to neglect the fact that chemotherapy also has serious limitations, often stemming from its failure to differentiate between normal and cancerous tissue, caused by the notorious toxicity of many of these chemotherapy drugs. Many patients recoil from chemo because of this simple fact.

I believe, however, it is possible to **make chemotherapy more effective and less toxic when it is given in certain innovative ways**. If someone close to me had cancer, and (after due deliberation) chemotherapy were deemed necessary, I would recommend looking into the innovative forms of delivering chemotherapy.

Innovative Forms of Chemotherapy

Low-dose Chemotherapy

Conventional chemotherapy (especially in the U.S.) is generally based on the principle of the maximum tolerated dose (MTD). This approach aims to administer high doses of cytotoxic drugs, the more, the better. Side effects tend to pile up, and so the MTD approach is typically followed by a rest period for the body to recover.

One of the most unexpected developments has been the realization that, while high-dose chemotherapy is harmful to the immune system, low doses of the same drugs can have the opposite effect. That is because they can decrease certain select populations of immunosuppressive subsets of cells. This is especially so with low doses of three specific drugs, oxaliplatin (Eloxatin®), cyclophosphamide (Cytoxan®), and gemcitabine (Gemzar®). (Shevchenko, Ivan, Svetlana Karakhanova, Sabine Soltek, Julia Link, Jagadeesh Bayry, Jens Werner, Viktor Umansky, and Alexandr V. Bazhin. "Low-Dose Gemcitabine Depletes Regulatory T Cells and Improves Survival in the Orthotopic Panc02 Model of Pancreatic Cancer." International Journal of Cancer 133, no. 1 (July 2013): 98–107; Chang, Li-Sheng, Wan-Lun Yan, Yu-Wen Chang, et al.Gemcitabine Enhances Antitumor Efficacy of Recombinant Lipoimmunogen-Based Immunotherapy. Oncoimmunology 5, no. 3 (March 2016): e1095433)

Background: Where did the idea of low-dose chemotherapy come from? Starting in the 1950s, the German cancer pioneer, Josef M. Issels, MD, used low-dose chemotherapy in his practice. He never proposed a mechanism for its action but empirically found it to be effective. Starting in the 1970s, another non-conventional pioneer, Ernesto Contreras, MD, used low-dose chemotherapy in his clinic in Tijuana, Mexico.

Low-dose Metronomic Chemotherapy

According to UpToDate.com, Metronomic chemotherapy uses frequent, lower doses of chemotherapy over long periods of time to target tumor angiogenesis [i.e., blood vessel growth] and minimize toxicity.

The NCI Cancer Dictionary expands on this definition:

"Treatment in which low doses of anticancer drugs are given on a continuous or frequent, regular schedule (such as daily or weekly), usually over a long time. Metronomic chemotherapy causes less severe side effects than standard chemotherapy. Giving low doses of chemotherapy may stop the growth of new blood vessels that tumors need to grow."

Metronomic chemotherapy has thus established a tiny beachhead in the world of chemotherapy. There are even scattered references to it in the NCCN guidelines. There are also at present over 700 articles in PubMed on the topic, with new ones appearing about once per week. About 100 of these refer to clinical trials, 25 of which are randomized controlled trials (RCTs). Clinicaltrials.gov lists ~25 trials currently recruiting patients. It is noteworthy that only one-quarter are from the United States, which was the birthplace and remains the bulwark of Maximum Tolerated Dose (MTD) chemotherapy.

IMMUNOTHERAPY

Immunotherapy has emerged as a game-changer in the fight against cancer. In recent years, a new class of immunotherapy drugs known as immune checkpoint inhibitors has taken center stage. Jim Allison, a pioneer in this field, invented Yervoy, the first immune checkpoint inhibitor, while at UC Berkeley. His groundbreaking work was recognized with the Nobel Prize in 2018.

The fundamental concept behind immune checkpoint inhibitors is to target the blocking factors produced by cancer cells and deactivate them. This action unleashes the body's immune system, enabling it to recognize and attack cancer cells with heightened vigor. The success of immune checkpoint inhibitors is particularly evident in melanoma, a life threatening form of skin cancer.

Combined treatment with two immune checkpoint inhibitors has exhibited significant efficacy in stage four melanoma patients. Approximately half of these patients experienced major responses, and around half of those achieved long-term remission. This achievement is unprecedented in the history of cancer treatment, especially for solid tumors in advanced stages. Jim Allison and other visionary scientists have spearheaded this groundbreaking advancement.

It is essential, however, to recognize that the effectiveness of immunotherapy varies among different cancer types and individuals. The key determinant of success is the tumor mutational burden (TMB). Cancers with higher mutation rates tend to respond better to immunotherapy, as the immune system detects abnormalities in these cells.

Specialized tests, such as Foundation Medicine's blood test and Memorial Sloan-Kettering's impact test, assess TMB and help identify suitable candidates for immunotherapy. Moreover, individual variations play a crucial role, as even cancer types traditionally considered unresponsive, like breast cancer, may show positive responses when exhibiting a high TMB.

Another critical factor influencing the success of immunotherapy is the absolute lymphocyte number, a component of the complete blood count (CBC) test. Patients with an absolute lymphocyte number of 1.8 or higher have a significantly greater chance of responding positively to immunotherapy. (Detailed information about absolute lymphocyte number and how to find yours is discussed earlier in this report). If this number falls below the threshold, interventions to boost the immune system become necessary before considering immunotherapy.

It is vital to ensure the immune system is in optimal condition before embarking on immunotherapy treatment. A robust immune system enhances the chances of a positive response to treatment. Strategies for achieving this include:

Nutritional Support: A diet rich in nutrient-dense natural whole foods form the foundation of immune system support.

Physical Activity: Regular, moderate exercise, such as brisk walking or swimming, plays a pivotal role in boosting the immune system and overall health.

Stress Management: Chronic stress weakens the immune system. Practices like meditation, deep breathing exercises, and yoga help manage stress levels and support immune function.

Supplementation: Immune-supportive probiotics and nutritional supplements, such as mushrooms, can complement efforts to strengthen the immune system.

It is also important to keep in mind that while immunotherapy offers remarkable promise, concerns have arisen regarding its toxicity, particularly with immune checkpoint inhibitors like Yervoy, Optivo, and Keytruda. These drugs can induce inflammation and adverse effects in various organs, making their use challenging. Innovative approaches are emerging to mitigate these issues, including:

Lower Doses: European practitioners are exploring lower doses of checkpoint inhibitors to reduce toxicity while maintaining efficacy.

Direct Tumor Injections: Injecting checkpoint inhibitors directly into tumors can enhance their effectiveness and minimize side effects.

Combination Therapies: Combining immunotherapy with viral therapies, such as Newcastle disease virus, or using common flu vaccines to "heat up" cold tumors shows promise in improving treatment outcomes.

Immunotherapy has ushered in a new era in cancer treatment, offering hope and promising results. While challenges exist, advancements in assessing TMB and the absolute lymphocyte number provide valuable tools for patient selection. Additionally, strategies to boost the immune system before treatment and innovative approaches to mitigate immunotherapy's toxicity are important to consider.

DEVELOPMENT OF TARGETED THERAPIES

Much cancer research has been a search for effective "targeted therapies." *What does 'targeted' mean in this context? Aren't all cancer drugs targeted to kill the cancer? Not exactly.* Classical chemotherapy is basically non-targeted, in that most of the original drugs killed rapidly dividing cells. This stemmed from the belief that cancers were characterized by a rapid redivision of malignant cells. This was true of the original targets of chemotherapy - acute leukemias, but not of the many slower growing cancers of adults.

Not all cancers are rapidly dividing, but many normal cells *do* divide rapidly. That is especially true of cells of the gastrointestinal (GI) tract, hair follicles and blood-forming system. That is why the typical side effects of chemotherapy are mouth sores, nausea and vomiting, hair loss and the general destruction of white blood cells.

The new generation of targeted drugs came to market in the 1990s, but originated much earlier. In the late 1930s, a Rochester, NY, physician named **A. Gordon Ide, MD** (1911-2003) was studying tumors transplanted into rabbits' ears. In addition to robust tumor growth, he observed a newly formed complex of veins and arteries. He was the first person to suggest that

tumors produced a substance that stimulated blood vessel growth. The observation was little noticed at the time.
(Ide AG, Baker NH, Warren SL. Vascularization of the Brown Pearce rabbit epithelioma transplant as seen in the transparent ear chamber. Am J Roentgenol 1939;42:891–899; http://obits.arizonagravestones.org/view.php?id=24365)

Then, in 1971, **Judah Folkman, MD** (1933-2008), a noted physician at Children's Hospital, Boston, isolated a "tumor angiogenic factor (TAF)" from extracts of cancer, and *"proposed that the growth of malignancies might be prevented if TAF activity were blocked."*
(Folkman, J. "Tumor Angiogenesis: Therapeutic Implications." The New England Journal of Medicine 285, no. 21 (November 18, 1971): 1182–86; see also: http://www.nature.com/focus/angiogenesis/classics/establish.html)

Folkman thought that it might be possible to target cancer's ability to create new blood supplies. He invented the term "angiogenesis inhibition" to describe this strategy, and began to experiment with substances that could block the formation of new blood vessels. The first such agents were derived from cartilage. This ability was eventually recognized as Hanahan and Weinberg's **cancer hallmark: sustained angiogenesis**.
(Brem, H., and J. Folkman. "Inhibition of Tumor Angiogenesis Mediated by Cartilage." The Journal of Experimental Medicine 141, no. 2 (February 1, 1975): 427–39)

Eventually, Folkman championed two substances that targeted new blood vessel formation. But although these drugs worked well in the laboratory, they never attained Food and Drug Administration (FDA) approval as drugs for humans.
(O'Reilly, M. S., T. Boehm, Y. Shing, N. Fukai, G. Vasios, W. S. Lane, E. Flynn, J. R. Birkhead, B. R. Olsen, and J. Folkman. "Endostatin: An Endogenous Inhibitor of Angiogenesis and Tumor Growth." Cell 88, no. 2 (January 24, 1997): 277–85; Wu, Z., M. S. O'Reilly, J. Folkman, and Y. Shing. "Suppression of Tumor Growth with Recombinant Murine Angiostatin." Biochemical and Biophysical Research Communications 236, no. 3 (July 30, 1997): 651–54)

Folkman was brilliant and accomplished, and his success in the laboratory led to a frenzy unparalleled in modern medical history. In particular, in May 1998, the *New York Times* ran a front-page story that raised the hopes of cancer patients worldwide. The Times' senior science reporter, Gina Kolata, wrote:

"Within a year if all goes well, the first cancer patient will be injected with two new drugs that can eradicate any type of cancer, with no obvious side effects and no drug resistance."
(Kolata, Gina. Hope in the lab: A special report.; A Cautious Awe Greets Drugs That Eradicate Tumors in Mice. New York Times, May 3, 1998)

Kolata quoted the Nobel laureate James D. Watson, PhD, co-discoverer of DNA's double helix, as saying, "Judah [Folkman] is going to cure cancer in two years." Kolata added:

"Dr. Watson said Dr. Folkman would be remembered along with scientists like Charles Darwin as someone who permanently altered civilization." (Ibid.)

When I visited Dr. Watson at Cold Spring Harbor in the summer of 2014 he was still fuming over the unauthorized quotes in this article.

Within days, the whole world had heard about Prof. Folkman's alleged "cure" for cancer. The ensuing frenzy sent the price of two pharmaceutical companies through the roof. The FDA promised quick approval. These names of Folkman's two drugs were **angiostatin** and **endostatin**. Never heard of them? No surprise, because both fizzled out almost as quickly as they had made headlines. In 2002, there were 88 PubMed-indexed articles on angiostatin. In 2017, there were just 13. Endostatin suffered a similar decline.

Folkman himself was not to blame for the fiasco. In fact he was quoted as saying, with self-deprecating humor: **"If you have cancer and you are a mouse, we can take good care of you."** (Ibid.) But he never claimed to have substances ready for human treatment.

It turned out, once again, that results achieved in laboratory mice did not readily translate into human clinical benefit. The whole episode had a profound effect on the future of cancer research. People were already challenging the logic behind conventional treatment. (My own book, *Questioning Chemotherapy*, had come out two years earlier.) *Folkman's work led to a search for drugs that could be more specific and therefore less toxic.*

Since this period also coincided with the Human Genome Project, it led to the development of drugs that were targeted against the growing panoply of genetic mutations associated with cancer. The era of 'targeted therapy' was thus born...also called "molecularly targeted drugs," "individualized treatment," "personalized" or "precision medicine."

There are now drugs that specifically target many of the most prominent genetic mutations within a tumor. These mutations, which are signposts of Hanahan and Weinberg's "Hallmarks of Cancer" allow cancers to grow, progress and metastasize.

The methods developed to establish the effectiveness of chemotherapy may not be relevant in assessing targeted therapies. Targeted therapies attack molecules associated with a particular person's cancer, while chemotherapy as a rule acts indiscriminately on all rapidly dividing cells. That is because targeted therapies are often "cytostatic," in that they block a tumor's proliferation, whereas conventional chemo is "cytotoxic" in that it kills rapidly-dividing cells.

Over the past 20 years, the FDA has approved many targeted therapies (with companion tests) to treat specific types of cancer. Even though the FDA still approves targeted therapies based on the anatomical location of the primary tumor (lung, breast, etc.), which was the pattern established for chemotherapy, *patients typically respond to targeted drugs if they have the genetic mutation in question, regardless of where the tumor first arose.*

In some cancers, one particular mutation predominates, and so it is more likely that a single targeted drug will be effective. In other cases, however, multiple targets appear in an unexpected pattern, and so genetic testing must be done to see which mutations predominate.

Genomic testing and treatments based on them have become a burgeoning subdivision of the industry. Many cancer centers have also jumped onto the precision medicine bandwagon. These include:

- Memorial Sloan-Kettering Cancer Center, New York, which uses a proprietary testing platform called MSK-ImpactTM (https://www.mskcc.org/blog/new-tumor-sequencing-test-will-bring-personalized-treatment-options-more-patients)
- City of Hope, previously known as Cancer Treatment Centers of America, Zion, IL; Tulsa, OK, Philadelphia, PA; Atlanta, GA; and Goodyear, AZ. They have made "precision medicine" a centerpiece of their treatment philosophy and hired an expert in the field, Maurie Markman, MD, as its President of Science and Medicine to help them make this transition to genomic medicine. (https://www.cancercenter.com/)
- The James Cancer Hospital of the Ohio State University, Columbus, OH https://cancer.osu.edu/locations/the-james-cancer-hospital-and-solove-research-institute
- The Mayo Clinic, Rochester, MN; Scottsdale and Phoenix, AZ; and Jacksonville, FL. The Mayo Clinic Health System also has dozens of locations in several states.

(https://www.mayoclinic.org/)

WHAT IS A RESPONSE?

There is a lot of confusion over what constitutes a "response" to cancer treatment. Yet this is often of paramount importance in trying to assess the comparative effectiveness of various treatment options.

The developers of new cancer treatments generally follow the "RECIST" criteria, which stands for "Response Evaluation Criteria in Solid Tumors." This is significant because "both tumor shrinkage (objective response) and time to the development of disease progression are important endpoints in cancer clinical trials."
Eisenhauer EA, Therasse P, Bogaerts J, et al. New response evaluation criteria in solid tumours: revised RECIST guideline (version 1.1). Eur J Cancer. 2009 Jan;45(2):228-47.)

There are four RECIST criteria (revised in 2009):

- Complete Response (CR): Disappearance of all lesions
- Partial Response (PR): At least a 30 percent decrease in the sum of the longest diameter of all lesions
- Stable Disease (SD): Neither sufficient shrinkage to qualify for a partial response nor sufficient increase to qualify for progressive disease
- Progressive Disease (PD): At least a 20 percent increase in the sum of the longest diameter of target lesions
- There is a debate in oncology over the significance of tumor shrinkages to the ultimate outcome of the treatment. The whole cancer drug marketplace ultimately rests on this issue. There is no question that responses, which are generally tumor shrinkages, are important in the early developmental stages of a new treatment. But early trials generally do not yield enough relevant information about the more meaningful survival of patients.

Do patients really live significantly longer by taking the treatment in question?

Randomized controlled (phase III) trials (RCTs), the so-called 'gold standard' of testing, are designed to yield information about survival. But, even here, there is disagreement over the most meaningful type of survival. There is a division of opinion between those who believe that progression-free survival (PFS) is the most important parameter, while others who argue—plausibly—that overall survival (OS) is more meaningful. It seems obvious that staying alive (with a good quality of life) is of paramount importance to most cancer patients. Plus, unlike PFS, overall survival is not dependent on anyone's subjective impression. The fact that people are alive or dead is easily established.

Which one does the U.S. Food and Drug Administration (FDA) favor, progression-free survival (PFS) or overall survival (OS)? It has vacillated on this question. The FDA used to require pharmaceutical companies to prove that a drug actually increased the test subjects' median overall survival. But after a while they began to grant accelerated approval based on increased responses or improvement in progression-free survival alone. In the case of the drug gemcitabine (Gemzar®), they even granted approval based solely on an improvement in quality of life.
(Belani CP, Eckardt J. Development of docetaxel in advanced non-small-cell lung cancer. Lung Cancer. 2004 Dec;46 Suppl 2:S3-11)

To gain approval, the drug manufacturer Eli Lilly worked with the FDA to create a new endpoint, which they termed "clinical benefit." This was designed to quantify the effect of their new drug on "patients' overall quality of life." It seemed obvious at the time that they did this because the drug did not have the desired effect on survival. To me, this seems like "moving the goalposts." In my discussion of various treatments, I will try to keep an eye on increases in median overall survival (OS) of all the patients in the treatment study group. But when this is impossible, as in the case of pilot studies, I will report tumor shrinkages and other benefits.

SIDE EFFECTS (ADVERSE EVENTS)

The issue of side effects is of critical importance in making a decision about treatment, since many treatments can have serious consequences in terms of both immediate (acute) and long-term (chronic) toxicity.

The U.S. government has devised a "severity scale" of side effects, which are now generally called "AEs," for adverse events. The government defines this as follows:

"An Adverse Event (AE) is any unfavorable and unintended sign (including an abnormal laboratory finding), symptom, or disease temporally associated with the use of a medical treatment or procedure...."
(The NCI Common Terminology Criteria for Adverse Events v4.0 (CTCAE). Publish Date: May 28, 2009. http://evs.nci.nih.gov/ftp1/CTCAE/CTCAE_4.03_2010-06-14_QuickReference_8.5x11.pdf)

There are five grades of AEs. As you investigate treatment options, you should pay attention to these criteria, for they give a clue as to what you might experience from any particular treatment. Everything in life has its pluses and minuses, and of course cancer treatments are no exception to this rule. There are often hidden "costs" of otherwise useful or even life-saving treatments.

- Grade 1: Mild; asymptomatic or mild symptoms; clinical or diagnostic observations only; intervention [i.e. treatment of the side effect] not indicated.
- Grade 2: Moderate; minimal, local or noninvasive intervention indicated; limiting age-appropriate instrumental ADL. [ADL = activities of daily living]
- Grade 3: Severe: medically significant but not immediately life-threatening; hospitalization or prolongation of hospitalization indicated; disabling; limiting self-care and ADL.
- Grade 4: Life-threatening; urgent intervention indicated.

CLINICAL TRIALS

- Clinical trials are of paramount importance in the cancer field.
- They are the indispensable linchpin of the drug approval process.
- They provide information that the FDA uses to determine the safety and efficacy of new drugs.
- They are the foundation of the $1 trillion pharmaceutical industry.
- They offer a treatment option for people with incurable cancers.

If "Big Pharma" (as the pharmaceutical industry is called) were a country, it would be larger than the economies of all but the 16 richest countries in the world—bigger than Turkey or the Netherlands, and twice as big as Austria or Thailand! When legislation is looming, The Pharmaceutical Industry can deploy an army of over 1,300 lobbyists to sway Congress with millions of dollars in campaign contributions. Big Pharma has bought and paid for thousands of experts who do its bidding in exchange for "honoraria," "speaking fees," and the like. Some of these payments may be legitimate, but many of them are thinly disguised bribes for favorable treatment.

Almost all pharmaceutical industry profits are based on the results of clinical trials. And because of the vast sums of money involved, "Big Pharma" ceaselessly promotes and defends the whole clinical trial system.

Frankly, Big Pharma influences the outcome of almost all major clinical trials. Headed by paid influencers (masquerading as impartial judges) these studies frequently exaggerate the benefits of drugs and downplay the frequency and severity of side effects. Paid promoters of the products of Big Pharma then invent ingenious arguments to justify outrageous prices, which for new cancer drugs are often set at $150,000 per patient per year. This is the cost of Merck's drug pembrolizumab (Keytruda®). According to the website of the Lown Institute:

"Keytruda has become a sales engine for Merck, making $4.5 billion in sales in the third quarter of 2021. Keytruda is close to becoming the highest-selling drug in the world and would be a Fortune 200 company on its own..."

Regulatory Capture

Despite periodic bouts of independence, regulatory agencies are under Big Pharma's sway. Regulatory capture was first described in the 1970s by the Nobel Prize economist, George Stigler. In one description it is *"a form of government failure which occurs when a regulatory agency, created to act in the public interest, instead advances the commercial or political concerns of special interest groups that dominate the industry or sector it is charged with regulating*." According to many commentators, the U.S. Food and Drug Administration (FDA) is a classic instance of a *"captured agency."*

Americans are divided along party lines on most issues. But the excessive cost of new drugs is one area of surprising unity. In a 2019 Kaiser Family Foundation poll, 79% of all Americans said that the price of new drugs was unreasonable. Sixty-three percent (63%) favored stricter government regulation on prices. This includes 80% of Republicans—traditionally opposed to regulation—who believe the government should negotiate with drug companies to get a lower price for people with Medicare.

NOTE: This sort of negotiation was included in the Inflation Reduction Act of 2022. The Act requires the Centers for Medicare & Medicaid Services (CMS) to negotiate the prices of certain prescription drugs under Medicare beginning in 2026.

We agree with these and other suggestions to rein in drug prices but we go much further. When it comes to cancer, we question the actual benefit that these new drugs provide. True scientists proceed from the "null hypothesis." They start from the premise that there is no significant difference between the specified groups in a clinical trial, and that any observed difference is due to sampling or experimental error. It is *the proponent's task* to prove that the treatment does work in a meaningful sense. Instead, today, in most big clinical trials, many of the key players are financially vested in achieving a positive outcome and act accordingly. As a result, it is an uphill battle, to put it mildly, to overcome their financial biases and get them to report the results in a truly impartial manner.

But are new cancer drugs as safe and effective as the great majority of people have been led to believe?

One major mission of *The Moss Report* is to cut through drug industry-inspired interpretations and achieve an unbiased assessment of the results. Unlike many reports written for the general public, we base our argument not on anecdotes, or emotion, but on facts that are revealed in the clinical trial papers themselves.

How Clinical Trials Work

Statements on the effects of new cancer drugs ultimately rest on the results of clinical trials. Drug companies (along with the National Institutes of Health, universities, and other nonprofit entities) advance proposed drugs through a series of laboratory and human experiments. The epitome of this process is the so-called "gold standard" of testing, the phase III randomized controlled trial (commonly abbreviated as RCT).

In a drug RCT, patients who have the same disease and other characteristics are randomly assigned to receive either an experimental agent or some other treatment. This other treatment may be another drug, a placebo (commonly called a "sugar pill"), or perhaps just best supportive care (BSC), in which a patient is made as comfortable as possible.

The reason for assigning patients at random (similar to the toss of a coin) is to eliminate any subjective bias in choosing who gets a particular treatment and who does not. There are myriad ways in an un-randomized trial that doctors can (consciously or unconsciously) influence the outcome. For instance, they may direct their healthier patients to the experimental drug, while consigning more advanced patients to the placebo group. This would prejudice the test in favor of the new drug.

First Clinical Trial

The idea of a clinical trial is ancient. There is a description of a primitive clinical trial in the 2nd century B.C.E. *Book of Daniel* (1:5-16). In this late Biblical account, Daniel convinced his jailers to feed him and his incarcerated colleagues a vegetarian diet, while giving some others a meat diet, and then to examine them for their impact on health:

"At the end of the ten days, Daniel and his three friends looked healthier and better nourished than the young men who had been eating the food assigned by the king."

Then the clinical trial went into eclipse for a few millennia. Next came James Lind's famous 1747 demonstration that lemons and limes would cure scurvy. But the randomized controlled trial (RCT) as we know it was created by a British statistician Austin Bradford Hill (1897-1991). Hill wrote an influential little book on the topic in the 1930s and along with a colleague conducted the first modern RCT in 1952. Patients were accepted into that trial based on well-defined criteria and were "randomly allocated to one of the treatment groups."

Today, the global clinical trials market has itself become a $44.2 billion behemoth (2018). In practice, only giant pharmaceutical companies ('Big Pharma") or organizations such as the U.S. government's National Institutes of Health (NIH) can afford to conduct or at least support full-scale testing.

NOTE: The U.S. government maintains a database of all current and many past clinical trials. It contains detailed descriptions of over 300,000 research studies, spanning all 50 states and 210 countries. There are ~90,000 trials specifically of cancer, of which ~47,000 are funded by academia; ~31,000 by industry, mainly "Big Pharma"; and ~13,000 by government agencies, mainly the NIH. Of the ~9,000 RCTs, the majority (~5,000) are funded either by industry or the NIH.

Regulatory agencies require the successful completion of phase III trials before they will allow the marketing of any new drug. The entire medical system is thus ultimately dependent on clinical trials. That is not to say that it is easy to buy one's way to approval. The system is rigorous and difficult. As of 2018, the probability of success of a new cancer drug stood at only **3.4%**. These were the drugs that made it all the way through the testing process and achieved final approval.

But we believe that even when a new drug does achieve approval, there are important reasons to question the validity of the claimed results.

FDA's "Accelerated Approval"

On its website, the FDA states:

"In 1992 FDA instituted the Accelerated Approval regulations. These regulations allowed drugs for serious conditions that filled an unmet medical need to be approved based on a surrogate endpoint. Using a surrogate endpoint enabled the FDA to approve these drugs faster."

"Surrogate endpoints may be used instead of clinical outcomes in some clinical trials. For example, surrogate endpoints are used when the clinical outcomes might take a very long time to study, or in cases where the clinical benefit of improving the surrogate endpoint is well understood. They are also used in cases where conducting a clinical endpoint study would be unethical. Before a surrogate endpoint can be accepted in place of a clinical outcome, extensive evidence must accumulate, including evidence from epidemiological studies and clinical trials. Usually clinical trials are needed to show that the surrogate endpoint can be relied upon to predict, or correlate with, clinical benefit in a context of use. Surrogate endpoints that have undergone this extensive testing are called validated surrogate endpoints and these are accepted by the FDA as evidence of benefit. Between 2010 and 2012, the FDA approved 45 percent of new drugs based on a surrogate endpoint. Sometimes surrogate endpoints can support an accelerated approval with lesser evidentiary support, when they are "reasonably likely to predict a clinical benefit"

Translation: The FDA's goal shifted to approving drugs faster rather than approving effective drugs in a reasonable amount of time!

Scholars who study these questions have emphasized the unpredictability of the relationship between progression-free survival (PFS) and overall survival (OS). According to the aforementioned government study:

"It is now recognized that the correlation between PFS and OS is both variable and unpredictable and depends on tumor type and tumor stage, as well as the particular drug being investigated....PFS is not always a reliable surrogate for OS...."

Who Decides on Quality of Life?

Another important point has to do with the assessment of the quality of life. Generally speaking, oncologists make the assessment on how the patient is feeling, regarding quality of life, not the patients themselves. Since oncologists frequently have a vested interest in the outcome of the trial, they have a motive to overstate how well the patient is feeling.

For example, when doctors and patients were each asked to evaluate the patient's performance status, they differed in the majority of cases (54%). And when the scores differed, in two-thirds of the cases (69%) the patients' rank claimed to have a worse performance status than the doctors did.

Industry-Sponsored Trials

It has frequently been noted that trials that are sponsored by industry have a greater likelihood of achieving positive results than those without such funding. For example, in a study of 159 randomized trials, it was found that:

"...the interpretation of the results of individual trials was significantly more favorable towards experimental interventions if funding was obtained from for-profit organizations."

Two systematic reviews found a similar kind of association between funding and pro-industry conclusions. For instance, Justin E. Beckelman and other scientists at Yale University School of Medicine, New Haven, published a large study on the topic in the *Journal of the American Medical Association (JAMA).* They noted the lack of research on this important topic:

"Despite increasing awareness about the potential impact of financial conflicts of interest on biomedical research, no comprehensive synthesis of the body of evidence relating to financial conflicts of interest has been performed."
(Bekelman JE, Li Y, Gross CP. Scope and impact of financial conflicts of interest in biomedical research: a systematic review. JAMA. 2003 Jan 22-29;289(4):454-65. doi: 10.1001/jama.289.4.454. PMID: 12533125)

Industry's Support of Research

The Yale authors noted that the drug and biotech industries' support of research in the U.S. increased dramatically, from 32% of such research in 1980 to 62% in 2000. At the same time, the federal government's share of research support fell, part of a more generalized trend towards privatization that followed the 1980 election of Ronald Reagan as president.

Whatever the alleged benefits of the shift toward privatizing drug and biotech industry research, this also resulted in "an **entanglement of relationships** among industry, investigators, and academic institutions also emerged."

One of the primary entanglements resulted in the development of a conflict of interest on the part of many researchers.

The authors of the above study defined a conflict of interests as:

"...a set of conditions in which professional judgment concerning a primary interest (such as a patient's welfare or the validity of research) tends to be unduly influenced by a secondary interest (such as financial gain)."

Their key findings were as follows:

- Approximately one-fourth of investigators had industry affiliations.
- Two-thirds of the academic institutions in question had a financial stake in start-ups sponsoring research at the same institutions.
- After evaluating a total of 1,140 original studies, there was "a statistically significant association between industry sponsorship and pro-industry conclusions."
- The odds ratio of reaching a positive conclusion when one has a financial stake in the outcome was rated as **3.6**. And for randomized controlled trials (RCTs) the odds ratio for a positive outcome was even higher, **4.14**.
- Industry sponsorship was also associated with restrictions on publication and data sharing.

The authors concluded:

"Financial relationships among industry, scientific investigators, and academic institutions are widespread. Conflicts of interest arising from these ties can influence biomedical research in

important ways."

You might ask, what is the harm in taking the industry's money, provided you reveal potential conflicts in advance? The reality is, although there is an occasional well-publicized 'slap on the wrists' for failure to disclose such ties, what is revealed is only the tip of the iceberg of industry penetration of the medical research community. For example:

"In 1997, approximately 16 percent of 1,396 highly ranked scientific journals had policies on conflicts of interest. Less than 1 percent of the articles published in these journals contained disclosures of personal financial interests."

Accurate Reporting?

In any discussion of adverse events, one assumes that the paper's authors report the side effects of treatment accurately. But researchers told the European oncology (ESMO) meeting in Copenhagen :

"A significant number of trials of targeted therapies...in recent years show suboptimal reporting of adverse events, particularly the reporting of recurrent or late toxicities and the duration of the adverse events...."

Scoring Poorly

According to Paolo Bossi, MD, of the Italian National Cancer Institute:

"**More than 90% of trials scored poorly** in their reporting of recurrent and late toxicities, and in reporting the duration of adverse events; 86% of trials did not adequately report on the time of the adverse event occurrence, and **75% of trials only reported on adverse events that occurred at a frequency above a fixed threshold**."

According to Nathan Cherny, MD, of Shaare Zedek Medical Center, Jerusalem, one reason for the underreporting of side effects is that editors rely on reports from doctors, not patients, about the frequency or severity of the side effects.

"[This] consistently leads to underreporting of adverse events and the severity of those events."

Therefore, we should take all reports of "minimal side effects" with a grain of salt. Such reports are frequently under-stated and under-reported.

Industry Control of Advisory Panels

How could a drug (such as another anti-lung cancer agent Iressa®) that showed "no benefit" in terms of response rates or time to progression or survival, still gain Food and Drug Administration (FDA) approval?

One answer lies in the cancer drug approval process itself. The FDA relies on advisory panels, which vote on whether or not to recommend approval of a therapy for the U.S. market. In cancer, the main panel is the Oncology Drug Advisory Committee (ODAC).

According to a July 2018 investigation by *Science* magazine, panel members are routinely questioned about potential biases before they vote on a drug. However, nothing is done to prevent drug company money from flowing to panelists *retroactively*. After key drug approval, the sponsoring company is free to shower money and other gifts to the panelists who approved the drug.

Science focused on the giant British-Swedish conglomerate AstraZeneca, and its billion-dollar heart drug, ticagrelor (Brilinta®). The findings were fully applicable to the cancer drug field as well.

The panelists all looked "clean" throughout the approval process. But after AstraZeneca achieved FDA approval for its drug, it made big payments to four members of the review panel. To quote the *Science* exposé:

"As Brilinta's sales took off later, however, AstraZeneca...showered the four with money for travel and advice. For example, those companies paid or reimbursed cardiologist Jonathan Halperin of the Icahn School of Medicine at Mount Sinai in New York City, ***more than $200,000*** *for accommodations, honoraria, and consulting from 2013 to 2016."*

These are just some of the ways that Big Pharma influences the outcome of a clinical trial and gains crucial FDA approval, even for an otherwise mediocre or dangerous drug.

Our general conclusion is that once approval is gained, drug companies rarely go back to see how well the same drugs would perform in the real world. A careful analysis of this one critical failure might throw doubt on a great many drugs that are considered safe and effective because of results obtained in phase II through III trials.

EVIDENCE-BASED MEDICINE

Think of evidence-based medicine (EBM) as a new chapter in an old book, where the plot suddenly shifts to give more voice to a character who had been in the background. In this narrative, you, the patient, are that character. Your complexities, your dreams, your needs—they all matter just as much as any laboratory test or clinical trial result. And it's about time, because medicine is not just a discipline of numbers and graphs. It's a discipline of people - living, breathing beings who laugh, cry, and love.

Imagine walking into a library filled with medical research, decades of doctors' experiences, and results from clinical trials around the world. Now imagine a guide who can sift through this enormous library and pick out only the most reliable, relevant, and proven information for you. That's essentially what Evidence-Based Medicine (EBM) does. It's a way for doctors to make sure they're offering you the best possible care by using treatments that have been thoroughly studied and found effective.

But here's the exciting part: This isn't just a one-way street where doctors dictate the terms. EBM has evolved. Today, it recognizes that you—the patient—also have crucial input to add. Think of it as customizing a suit or a dress. The tailor knows the craft inside and out, but you're the one who'll be wearing it, so your style and comfort matter just as much. Similarly, EBM combines the best scientific evidence with your own preferences, beliefs, and lifestyle to create a cancer treatment plan tailored just for you.

This is a big deal. It marks a shift towards a more 'patient-centered' approach in medicine. Your opinions, philosophies, and even your personal goals for treatment are considered valid pieces of evidence that can guide the decision-making process. It's a partnership between you and your healthcare team, built on a foundation of trust, respect, and shared knowledge.

The next time you're in a conversation with your healthcare provider, remember: You're not just a spectator; you're a critical player. And with the support of EBM, you're both drawing from the best knowledge available to make well-informed decisions about your care.

The Three Pillars of EBM

- **Best Available Evidence:** This includes the latest research, clinical guidelines, and expert opinions.

- **Clinical Expertise:** The judgment and experience of healthcare professionals in applying evidence to individual patients.
- **Patient Values and Preferences:** Recognizing that patients' beliefs, goals, and desires play a vital role in decision-making.

Examples and Application

- **Shared Decision Making:** This approach involves clinicians and patients working together to make decisions, weighing medical evidence and personal values. For example, a patient with early-stage prostate cancer might choose active surveillance over surgery, considering both the statistical outcomes and their own quality of life priorities.
- **Informed Consent:** Beyond just a form to sign, true informed consent means understanding all available options, the evidence behind them, and how they align with personal values.
- **Chronic Disease Management:** For conditions like diabetes, individual lifestyle preferences, cultural dietary habits, and personal goals must be integrated with evidence-based guidelines to create an effective and sustainable care plan.

The Changing Role of Healthcare Providers

- **From Authority to Guide:** The doctor isn't just an authority figure prescribing a one-size-fits-all treatment but acts as a guide, helping patients navigate the complex landscape of modern healthcare.
- **Empathy and Communication:** Building trust, understanding patient values, and effective communication are as crucial as medical expertise.

In a world where we're often reduced to numbers and statistics, the recognition of personal philosophies and preferences within Evidence-Based Medicine (EBM) is a breath of fresh air. It signals a transformation in healthcare that's nothing short of revolutionary. This isn't just about blending hard scientific data with a patient's own beliefs and lifestyle choices; it's also about restoring a 'human touch' to medicine—a field often criticized for its clinical detachment.

By welcoming patient input and perspective into the decision-making process, this evolved model of EBM doesn't just acknowledge that medical outcomes are about individuals; it also recognizes that those individuals bring their own rich tapestries of experiences and values to the table. This blend of scientific rigor and personal insight creates a healthcare landscape where empathy and collaboration are not just buzzwords but guiding principles.

Ultimately, this transformative shift toward a more compassionate and inclusive healthcare system reminds us that the essence of medicine has always been a delicate dance between science and the human spirit. And in this dance, both partners are finally learning to move in greater harmony.

CHOOSING CARE

PERSONALIZED HEALTHCARE

Empowering patients through understanding is a cornerstone of personalized healthcare. It goes beyond merely relaying medical terms; it's about offering a nuanced understanding of the disease, the treatments available, and how they interact within the individual's unique biological framework.

Knowledge Is Power: A well-informed patient isn't just a passive recipient of medical care; they become an active participant in their own healing journey. When patients understand the underlying mechanisms of their disease and the intended effects of their treatments, they're better positioned to make choices that align with their goals and values.

Individualized Journey: Cancer is not a one-size-fits-all disease. Each type and stage comes with its own set of challenges and treatment options. By gaining a deep understanding of the specific type and stage of cancer they're facing, patients can collaborate more effectively with healthcare providers to customize a treatment plan that is both scientifically sound and personally meaningful.

Strengths of Conventional Treatment: Traditional medical approaches, including surgery, radiation, chemotherapy, and targeted therapies, have undergone rigorous scientific testing and have shown effectiveness in treating a wide array of cancer types. These treatments often serve as the cornerstone of oncological care, shrinking tumors, eliminating cancerous cells, and improving survival rates.

Limitations: However, it's crucial to understand that conventional treatment methods are not without their drawbacks. They can come with an array of side effects ranging from fatigue and nausea to more severe complications like organ damage. Moreover, each individual's biological makeup, the specific type and stage of cancer, and other health factors can significantly influence the effectiveness of conventional treatments.

Complementary Approaches: For those looking to augment their conventional treatment plan, various complementary therapies offer additional routes to enhance well-being. Nutrition, physical therapy, and mindfulness practices, among others, can help manage side effects, improve emotional resilience, and optimize overall health. While they are not intended to replace conventional treatments, these approaches can offer a more holistic way to manage cancer, targeting not just the disease but the person as a whole.

GETTING THE BEST POSSIBLE CARE

The relationship between professional care and self-help is delicate. It requires mutual respect and understanding from both the doctor and the patient. Doctors believe in evidence-based medicine, but the evidence for or against complementary treatments is often patchy or inadequate. This is where the old dictum, *"Above all, do no harm,"* comes into play.

It is important to draw clear boundaries between professional care and self-help. This will ensure that you get the best possible care without infringing on either patient autonomy or medical expertise.

The domain of professional care includes:

- **Expertise:** Medical professionals are trained to diagnose, treat, and manage health conditions. They have access to diagnostic tools and specialized knowledge.
- **Ethics:** Medical ethics governs professional practice, ensuring that the welfare of the patient is prioritized.
- **Limitations:** Recognizing the value of patients' insights and experiences and incorporating them into the care plan.

The domain of self-help includes:

- **Autonomy:** Patients have the right to make choices about their care and to seek alternative or complementary treatments.
- **Personal responsibility:** Engaging in healthy lifestyle choices and being proactive in

managing one's health.

- **Limitations:** Recognizing the importance of professional medical advice, especially in complex or critical health situations.

The balance between professional medical care and self-help requires ongoing communication, trust, and respect. Both parties should acknowledge the importance of each other's roles while recognizing the limitations, ensuring a partnership that honors the complexity and individuality of health and well-being.

A NOTE ON INTEGRATIVE CARE

Like medical oncology itself, the field of complementary and alternative medicine (CAM) requires expert and specialized input. Let me reiterate my belief that **cancer patients, whenever possible, should be under the care of both highly trained oncologists and also excellent CAM practitioners.**

These practitioners should be licensed in their respective states or countries, or if not, then working under the supervision of a licensed medical doctor. They should be integrated as much as possible into the patient's team of caregivers. True integration is a reality in a few hospitals and clinics, but is still an aspiration in most places. So the patient may need to assemble his or her own team of experts and to weave together the various components as best as possible.

CHOOSING A HOSPITAL

There is no objective way of determining the very best cancer doctors and hospitals. Obviously, there can be outstanding doctors at mediocre hospitals, and vice versa. Start with the U.S. News rankings of hospitals for both cancer and any other relevant subspecialty. U.S. News also lists, but does not rank, specialists in various areas. Look in particular for experienced doctors at top-rated centers that have a high safety rating. All other things being equal, I try to choose doctors who are **mid-way in their careers** and are therefore likely to offer a good blend of experience and capability.

One problem you will quickly discover is that there is generally an inverse relationship between the reputation of a physician or surgeon and the speed within which you can get into his or her practice. The doctor you may want may be the hardest to get—because many others are going through the same decision-making process. You may then need to compromise and take the doctor's associate, who is less busy.

Your primary care doctor or specialist may make a recommendation to a local colleague. But many people do not realize that their health insurance (including Medicare) will often pay for conventional care at top-rated U.S. hospitals, regardless of their location. (Unfortunately, this does not usually apply to complementary and alternative medicine).

This raises the difficult question of whether or not to seek treatment exclusively within your home area, to travel to a regional center, or to go to the best center of excellence, even if that means traveling to a distant city, with all the costs and difficulties that may entail. This often comes down to a question of money. Usually you will have a better outcome if you go to the best possible hospital, regardless of its location.

IMPORTANT DECISIONS

We cannot emphasize enough how important it is to choose wisely in this regard. Dealing with a cancer diagnosis is one of life's most challenging moments. Oftentimes, there is an atmosphere of panic surrounding the decisions, especially if oncologists and others are telling you that you must make your decision immediately. However, there is an equally compelling reason to do your research. A successful outcome oftentimes relates to the skill, experience, and sanitary practices of the doctors, nurses, and ancillary staff.

Go to an Experienced Center

Treatment of cancer requires the thorough and precise examination of the patient to determine the exact nature and extent of the disease. A doctor's experience is also decisive. While the National Comprehensive Cancer Network (NCCN) guidelines call for patients with cancer to receive treatment at centers with expertise, it was for a long time unknown just how beneficial this was.

An analysis of institutions with high volume vs. low volume found that, after accounting for differences in the radiotherapy protocols, **patients treated in high-volume centers had longer overall survival vs. patients treated at low-volume institutions**.

Benefits of Large, Experienced Hospitals

Major cancer hospitals have mortality rates (deaths of patients under their care) under 5%. Nationwide, major complications occur in 10% to 20% of patients, and some sort of complication occurs in about 40%. Recovery time may take up to one year. Major complications include respiratory or cardiovascular complications and clinically apparent "anastomotic leak" (i.e., a breakdown along a surgical connection of two structures, an anastomosis, which causes fluids to leak).

A study from Holland also showed a huge difference in outcome between what are called high-volume and low-volume centers in Europe as well:

"Mortality and morbidity rates [for one kind of cancer] were significantly lower in the high-volume center, which had in-hospital mortality of 5% vs 13%....hospital volume...proved to be strong prognostic factors predicting in-hospital mortality...For stage I and stage II disease, there was a significantly better five-year survival in the high-volume center."
(Wouters, Michael W., Bas P. Wijnhoven, Henrieke E. Karim-Kos, et al. "High-Volume versus Low-Volume for Esophageal Resections for Cancer: The Essential Role of Case-Mix Adjustments Based on Clinical Data." Annals of Surgical Oncology 15, no. 1 (January 2008): 80–87)

Many people just take the treatment offered to them at their local hospital. This is the most convenient course and, of course, traveling does entail the extra cost of hotel rooms and meals for any companion. But patients may not realize that their insurance will often pay for medical treatment at "centers of excellence." True, the travel expenses and hotel costs in a nearby city can be considerable. But one must compare the costs to reducing the chance of dying from the procedure itself from 13% to 5% or lower at the most experienced medical centers.

What constitutes sufficient "experience"? A study in the *Journal of Clinical Oncology* showed that this is associated with what is called "change points," which are the points at which measurably better or worse results are attained. At **15 particular operations**, the 30-day mortality rate (within which death is presumed to have occurred as a result of the operation itself) **decreased from 7.9% to 3.1%**—less than half. Later "change points" are 35 operations and 59 operations. These were both associated with improvements in one-, three-, and five-year survival rates.

Seek out the best medical care available for the treatment of your condition, even if that means traveling for treatment. When your life hangs in the balance, if you can, make the trip and accept the extra cost and inconveniences that come with it. The record shows that it matters in terms of the ultimate outcome.

These three resources will help narrow your search for excellent and safe health care providers in any given U.S. locale:

- *U.S. News*
- Medicare.gov
- The Leapfrog Group

Using these three, you can come to a good understanding of the quality and safety of the health opportunities available to you either in your locale or at a distance from your home.

U.S. News

US News and World Report publishes a ranking of the top U.S. hospitals. You can find this readily enough on the Internet. Pick your hospital wisely and don't jump at the most convenient one. This website offers detailed information on a hospital's general background, history, and specific information on particular doctors, including ranking them. As they state,

"U.S. News has extensive information in each doctor's profile to help you find the best one for you."

For example, we chose a particular doctor we know at Memorial Sloan-Kettering Cancer Center, a man with a well-deserved national and international reputation. We were surprised to learn that he had only a "fair" rating (two out of five stars) from his patients, based on 36 reviews!

We then looked up another doctor we knew at NYU Langone Medical Center in New York. He got five out of five stars, based on 39 reviews. This corresponded with our experience with him.

But in other cases, we vehemently disagreed with these patient evaluations. It left us wondering if some ambitious doctors hadn't learned how to "game the system," by manipulating patients (or others) to leave positive 5-star reviews.

Medicare's Hospital Compare

A U.S. government website "Hospital Compare" also offers good insight into the quality of various hospitals. It allows you to directly compare hospitals in a particular locale, although, unfortunately, not specifically for any particular kind of cancer. Gauge the record in other critical areas to reach a conclusion on their general record of effectiveness and safety.

Medicare gives an overall rating and, often, a very useful patient survey rating which measures patients' experiences of their own hospital care:

"Recently discharged patients were asked about important topics like how well nurses and doctors communicated, how responsive hospital staff was to their needs, and the cleanliness and quietness of the hospital environment."

This website also tells American patients how far away the hospital is from their ZIP code, offers a chance to like or save the reference to a particular facility, and to compare it to other facilities. Even more detailed information, including the ranking of each facility compared to the national average for mortality, safety of care, the readmission rate, patient experience, effectiveness of care, timeliness of care, and efficient use of medical imaging.

Under the "Patient Survey Rating" category, one finds information on the following (with data comparing it to the U.S. national average): Patients reported that:

- Their nurses always communicated well.

- Their doctors always communicated well.
- They always received help as soon as they wanted.
- Their room and bathroom were always clean.
- The staff always explained about medicines before giving it to them.
- The area around their room was always quiet at night.
- They were given information about what to do during their recovery at home.
- They understood their care when they left the hospital.
- They gave their hospital a rating of 9 or 10 on a scale from 0 (lowest) to 10 (highest).
- They would definitely recommend the hospital to a friend or loved one.

Additional detailed information on the following:

- Timely and effective care
- Complications and deaths
- Unplanned hospital visits
- Psychiatric unit services
- Payment and value of care

Comparing Search Engines for Care Centers, an Example

Within 100 miles of Blue Hill, Maine, for example, Medicare.gov found 13 hospitals with a four-star rating. (There were none with a five-star rating.) The closest hospital was Northern Light Blue Hill Memorial Hospital, which got an overall rating of 4 stars. This was based on how well it performs in different indicators of quality, including the treatment of heart attacks, pneumonia, readmission rates, and safety of care. Overall, this seemed too optimistic for such a small town.

When we filtered the results to show only facilities with both a four or five-star rating and an identical patient rating there was only one such facility: Pen Bay Medical Center in Rockport. But, according to LeapFrog, Pen Bay is only a "Top Rural Hospital." That's a good ranking for what it represents, but it is hardly a center of excellence for complicated cancer surgery or other treatments. **Overall, we would rely on the U.S. News and Leapfrog algorithms rather than Medicare.gov to make consequential decisions about medical treatment facilities.**

Leapfrog Hospital Survey

Since surviving treatment for your cancer is critically important, pay special attention to the safety record, not just of any particular treatment, but of each institution that you are considering. Another website that is very helpful at determining this is called Leapfrog Hospital Survey: 2,200 hospitals provide data for this survey. The emphasis is on improving the safety record of American hospitals.

Leapfrog provides a very handy Leapfrog Hospital Safety Grade. This is the only hospital rating that is focused exclusively on safety. It's A, B, C, D, or F letter grades are "a quick way for consumers to choose the safest hospital to seek care." Here is a good description of this admirable project:

"The background is that 200,000+ Americans die annually due to preventable mistakes in hospitals, according to the Journal of Patient Safety. To draw attention to this epidemic, in 2012

The Leapfrog Group decided to expand its focus beyond employers to reach consumers directly. Out of this vision came the Leapfrog Hospital Safety Grade, a letter grade rating of how safe hospitals are for patients. The Safety Grade provides consumers with the critical information on how likely they are to experience accidents, injuries, errors or harm while in the hospital."

Leapfrog provides data on:

Practices for safer health care, including hand hygiene, nursing workforce, a culture of safety, leadership pertaining to safety, and teamwork training

- Safe surgical volumes for high-risk surgeries
- ICU staffing to reduce mortality
- Infection rates for hospital-acquired infections
- Hospitals' Never Events policies
- Use of bar code technology to reduce medication errors

HELPING YOURSELF

COMMUNICATION AND COLLABORATION

Team Effort: Conquering cancer is not a one-person job, nor is it solely the responsibility of your medical team. Successful treatment is often the result of a collaborative approach, where the practitioners and the patient work together in concert. Each party brings unique insights and skills to the table. The medical team provides expertise and professional guidance, while the patient brings their lived experience, preferences, and the will to fight and recover.

Open Dialogue: Navigating cancer treatment is a complex journey, and understanding each step can empower you to make the best choices for your health. Don't hesitate to ask questions, express your concerns, or seek a deeper understanding of your treatment plan from your medical team. Knowing the rationale behind a specific treatment or medication can help demystify the medical jargon and alleviate some of the natural apprehension that comes with battling cancer.

Appointment Companions: Given the often complex and emotionally charged nature of medical appointments, it's highly beneficial to bring a family member, friend, or caregiver with you. This extra set of ears can help catch details you might miss, ask questions you might not think of, and provide emotional support during what can be an intense experience.

AN INTRODUCTION TO THE MOSS METHOD™

As discussed earlier in **The Hallmarks of Cancer**, Dr. Moss has identified three crucial areas where patients can take steps to help themselves. Lifestyle changes can make a difference. This approach involves the use of specific foods, supplements, herbs, and other approachable and gentle actions. It is as safe and manageable as one can find in the complex realm of cancer care. But its real strength is its foundation on important scientific discoveries.

CANCER STEM CELLS (CSC'S)

CSC's are responsible for the Progression and metastasis of cancer

To paraphrase Hanahan and Weinberg's brilliant but highly technical explanation, cancer cells are the starting point of the disease and are responsible for making it worse. They carry the specific genetic changes that make cancer what it is. For a long time, people thought that most cancer cells in a tumor were pretty much the same until the disease got really advanced. At that point, the cancer cells would start to differ from each other, leading to different types or 'clones' of cancer cells within the same tumor. This is why, under a microscope, many tumors look like a mixed bag of cells with different features, such as levels of growth, blood supply, and inflammation. However, recent research has shown that tumors are more complex than we thought. There is now evidence for a special type of cancer cell within tumors, called 'cancer stem cells,' which adds another layer of complexity to the disease.

Here are some of the characteristics of cancer stem cells:

- They can make copies of themselves, creating more stem cells just like them.
- They can turn into different kinds of cancer cells that make up the tumor.
- They often shrug off common treatments like chemo and radiation.
- They're the "travelers" of the cancer world, more likely to spread the disease to other body parts.

Even though we're still sorting through and piecing together this information, we know that cancer stem cells (CSCs) are found in many tumors, although in varying amounts. The cancers in which they have been found include:

- Leukemia (both acute and chronic types)
- Breast Cancer
- Colorectal Cancer
- Lung Cancer (both non-small cell and small cell types)
- Prostate Cancer
- Glioblastoma (a type of brain cancer)
- Ovarian Cancer
- Pancreatic Cancer
- Liver Cancer (hepatocellular carcinoma)
- Melanoma (skin cancer)
- Head and Neck Squamous Cell Carcinoma
- Multiple Myeloma
- Further examples are being discovered.

What makes CSCs special is their ability to start new tumors, initially seen in lab rodents. Often, these cells also carry specific markers, similar to the regular stem cells from where the cancer started. This presents a problem since vaccines and other treatments that target these markers might also interfere with vital normal functions.

Cancer Stem Cell research is an exciting frontier in oncology. In our opinion, the pioneers of this field, including Profs. John Dick of Toronto and Max Wicha of the University of Michigan, among others, deserve a Nobel Prize for this work. Recently, scientists have been delving deeper into understanding CSCs and their unique role in the growth and spread of tumors. This research is opening doors to potential new treatments that specifically target these cells, offering hope for more effective and tailored cancer therapies.

Building on the insights gained from studying CSCs, scientists are not only reshaping our understanding of cancer's complexity but also igniting optimism about the future of cancer treatment. As the field progresses, the potential to revolutionize oncology by harnessing the power of this knowledge is enormous, bringing us closer to a world where advanced cancer is more manageable, or possibly curable.

Interestingly, researchers have found that some natural substances can target cancer stem cells (CSCs) across different types of tissue. In Pittsburgh, a city with a long history in cancer research, **scientists have posited that the real issue in cancer may not be the rapidly dividing cells we usually focus on, but rather the stem cells that birth them.** This could explain why many cancers come back even after initial treatments seem successful. These treatments might be missing the root cause: dormant cancer stem cells that escape eradication.

Researchers are actively pursuing this line of inquiry not only in Pittsburgh but also in California, Texas, New York, and numerous labs globally.

In *The Moss Method™*, we emphasize eating foods and taking supplements that have been shown to specifically target CSCs, without harming normal cells.

One standout is curcumin, the yellow component of turmeric, a root commonly used in Asian cuisine. Studies, including those from the University of Michigan, suggest that when curcumin is paired with piperine, a compound in black pepper, it can halt or even reverse the growth of dangerous CSCs. And it does so without harming our regular, healthy cells. Curcumin is part of a group of natural compounds in foods proven to target CSCs, and considering the low risks involved, these easily accessible food-based elements offer significant promise.

For deeper insight into curcumin and other cancer, read our companion book, *The Moss Method: Fight Cancer Naturally.*

CANCER AS A METABOLIC DISEASE

Cancer is Characterized by Disordered Metabolism

Think of your body as a bustling city where energy is the currency that keeps everything running smoothly. Just like a city needs roads and power sources, your cells need energy to function properly. This energy comes from metabolism, a complex process that converts food into fuel. However, sometimes, this energy system goes awry, and cancer can be a result.

Now imagine Otto Warburg as an early detective in this mystery. Back in the 1920s, he noticed that *cancer cells* seemed to have a different way of producing energy. They preferred a high-octane fuel called glucose, even when plenty of oxygen was around. This unusual behavior came to be known as the "Warburg effect."

This concept was given little credence until modern medicine took Warburg's old ideas to the next level with FDG-PET scans. These scans use a special dye that light up areas of the body with high glucose uptake, helping doctors spot potential cancer hotspots. About 90% of all cancerous tumors will light up on an FDG-PET scan.

Here's where you can take charge. Scientists have also found that certain lifestyle changes can influence how cancer cells get their energy. A low-carb ketogenic style diet is one approach. By cutting down on sugars and carbs, you're making it tougher for cancer cells to thrive on their preferred energy source. Additionally, practicing intermittent fasting is like hitting pause on their mealtime – it gives normal cells a chance to repair, while making it harder for cancer cells to get the energy they need.

Depriving cancer cells of energy is like outsmarting a crafty opponent. It's a self-help strategy where you take control of your body's energy system, making it less friendly for cancer cells. While it's not a standalone treatment, combining these lifestyle changes with medical therapies can create a more challenging environment for cancer to grow.

So, while the relationship between metabolism and cancer is complex, you can be the hero of your own story. By understanding how cancer cells use energy differently, you can make smart choices about diet and lifestyle, helping to create a less welcoming environment for them. In this battle, knowledge truly is power – your power to take control and support your body's natural defenses!

THE IMMUNE SYSTEM & CANCER

A Major Function of the Human Immune System is to Kill and Control Cancer Cells

Patients with a robust immune system have a better chance of long-term disease-free survival than those with weakened immunity. There are self-help ways derived from traditional medicine to boost the immune system and stop the spread of cancer.

Our **immune system** is always working to protect us from harmful invaders, such as microbes, but also cancer cells. It's a network of special cells and proteins that help keep us healthy. Sometimes, though, cancer can develop. This happens when our cells start to grow out of control and form a lump (called a tumor), or so-called 'liquid tumors' called leukemia, lymphoma or myeloma.

But here's the good news: our immune system doesn't give up easily. It's always on the lookout for anything that shouldn't be there, including cancer cells. It has its own set of super-powered cells called T cells that can recognize and attack these rogue cells. However, cancer cells can sometimes be tricky and hide from the immune system's radar.

Increasingly, scientists and doctors are working together to help the immune system fight cancer better and develop immunotherapy treatments that give the immune system a boost so it can target and destroy cancer cells more effectively. These treatments help make the body's own immune system stronger and smarter in its battle against cancer.

It's been a long slog to get here. The roots of immune-based cancer treatments go way back to the work of pioneers like William B. Coley, MD, in the late 1800s. Coley, a largely unsung hero, noticed that some cancer patients who also had a particular kind of bacterial infection, seemed to fare much better than average. He developed "Coley's toxins," which were mixtures of killed bacteria that sometimes triggered fevers and a powerful response to cancer. While his methods were ahead of his time, and never resulted in a proper clinical trial, they laid the foundation for future research.

In more recent decades, scientists such as the National Cancer Institute's Steven A. Rosenberg, MD and Memorial Sloan Kettering's Lloyd J. Old, MD (one of Dr. Moss's early mentors) made groundbreaking strides in understanding how the immune system could be harnessed to fight cancer. Rosenberg's work with T cells and Old's research on tumor necrosis factor (TNF) and numerous other accomplishments paved the way for today's innovative treatments.

As a result, immunotherapy has finally become the "fourth modality" in cancer treatment (after surgery, radiation and chemotherapy). With ongoing research and breakthroughs, doctors continue to develop innovative ways to unleash the full power of the immune system against cancer. Imagine a world where we can use our body's natural defenses to fight cancer without harsh side effects. This means gentler and more effective treatments, and even the possibility of preventing cancer from coming back.

While cancer is admittedly a tough opponent, science is definitely on our side. By strengthening our immune system and giving it the tools it needs, we're edging closer to a future where we can beat cancer with optimism and hope. We have a super power: our own immune system.

TOGETHER, THESE FUNDAMENTAL APPROACHES MAKE UP *THE MOSS METHOD™*

The Moss Method™ is a powerful way to fight cancer, naturally. In the journey to conquer cancer, this self-help approach can be a game-changer. *The Moss Method™*, comprising three dynamic elements, opens up new avenues for cancer "healers" to take proactive and beneficial steps in the fight against cancer. These elements – targeting cancer stem cells, attacking disordered metabolism, and harnessing the immune system – present a unique opportunity to contribute positively to one's own health journey, without conflicting with conventional oncology.

First, by understanding and targeting cancer stem cells, you're addressing the root cause of cancer's growth and recurrence. Armed with knowledge about natural compounds, foods, and supplements, you can create a less hospitable environment for these resilient cells, potentially slowing down their progress.

Second, the disordered metabolism of cancer cells offers a target that can be affected by lifestyle choices. Embracing a low-carb, ketogenic style diet and practicing intermittent fasting can alter the energy landscape, depriving cancer cells of their preferred fuel source and potentially making treatments more effective.

Finally, the immune system, our body's natural defense mechanism, holds immense potential. Boosting it through various means, like immunotherapy and lifestyle adjustments for a healthy microbiome, can enhance its ability to recognize and eliminate cancer cells.

The Moss Method™ brings these three aspects together, empowering you with options that can complement the work of medical professionals. By incorporating self-help measures that align with these pillars, you're not only being proactive in your journey but also contributing to a comprehensive strategy to battle cancer from multiple angles.

It's important to remember that *The Moss Method™* is not a standalone solution. Rather, it's a supportive strategy that complements conventional treatments, offering a holistic approach to cancer care. By embracing these elements, you're not only advocating for your own well-being but also actively participating in your healing journey. In this collective effort, science, medical expertise, and self-empowerment converge, laying the foundation for healing.

ADDITIONAL RESOURCES

We know it is important for some readers to pursue their own research on cancer. *What are the best resources for doing so?* The U.S. government's **PubMed** is the go-to source for all 28 million medical research articles that have been indexed. Every search begins and ends at http://www.ncbi.nlm.nih.gov/ pubmed/ (or simply type pubmed.com into your browser and it will transfer you there).

When it comes to conventional treatment recommendations, the most definitive source is the **National Comprehensive Cancer Network (NCCN).** This is a project of 27 leading American cancer centers to harmonize the treatment of almost every type of cancer. Each section is written by a panel of academic experts and recommendations are put into four categories, based upon the strength of these recommendations and the degree of unanimity among the reviewers.

There are several limitations to the NCCN for the average reader, however. First, the language employed is very technical and thus the recommendations may be difficult to understand. Second, there are often so many possible alternatives that one faces "paralysis by analysis." Third, the core of NCCN is a set of nomograms, or diagrams, rather than a narrative. Non-scientists may have difficulty interpreting these. Nonetheless, the NCCN reports are the 'blueprints' that increasingly guide cancer treatment decisions at conventional clinics around the world. There is also a corresponding set of reports for lay people. These overcome the above problems but, alas, are too simplified to be of use to serious readers. You must sign up to use NCCN, but it is open to non-physicians and is free. (https://www.nccn.org/professionals/physician_gls/f_guidelines.asp#site)

Another important source of information available to all cancer patients is the 'professional level' statements of the *National Cancer Institute's* **Physicians' Data Query (PDQ)** database (www.cancer.gov). Generally, they do a pretty good job. Again, you should attempt to utilize the health professional statements of this website and ignore the too-simplified statements written for lay people.
(http://www.cancer.gov/types)

One of the best fee-based resources on cancer is a searchable compendium of medical textbooks, the **LWW Health Library**. This is a subscription-based service that simultaneously accesses the textbooks of the medical publisher, Wolters Kluwer. A subscription includes online access to the most widely quoted of all cancer textbooks, DeVita, Hellman and Rosenberg's *Cancer: Principles and Practice of Oncology* (12th edition, Philadelphia: Walter Kluwers, 2023, with quarterly online updates. Sometimes the opinions of the DeVita authors will clarify the choices offered by the NCCN. The DeVita chapters are supposed to be updated throughout the course of the year by expert reviewers. However, I find that these updates are of uneven quality. Some are skimpy or infrequent. Nonetheless, this is an outstanding resource that every serious student of cancer needs to have.

Another outstanding resource is **UpToDate.com**. Thoroughly edited by leading physicians, this is a subscription service at $495 per year. It also deals with many other diseases and conditions, but is particularly strong in cancer. UpToDate is easier to use than NCCN. Because it generally lives up to its name, and has an equally distinguished group of authors as DeVita, I find that I frequently use this as my "go to" source on conventional treatment options. Some libraries may provide you with access at no cost.

GETTING READY FOR YOUR JOURNEY

Being equipped with comprehensive knowledge and a nuanced understanding of your medical condition serves as more than just a psychological comfort—it's a potent tool for decision-making. Informed patients are better positioned to make choices that align with their personal values, lifestyle, and ultimate objectives. Whether one opts for aggressive treatments or focuses on preserving quality of life is a highly individual decision, shaped by a multitude of factors ranging from familial responsibilities to personal philosophies on life and mortality.

The cancer journey transcends clinical procedures and protocols; it's a profoundly human experience demanding emotional fortitude, proactive involvement, and an unswerving focus on the individual at its core. Comprehending the complexities of cancer and its treatments not only demystifies a labyrinthine process but also empowers patients to regain some semblance of control. Ultimately, it's not just about being a patient; it's about being an empowered individual confronting a substantial life challenge.

Disclaimer

Ralph W. Moss, Ph.D. Is Not a Medical Doctor

Ralph W. Moss earned a doctor of philosophy degree from Stanford University (1974) and has been a medical journalist in the cancer field since that time, beginning with his time at Memorial Sloan-Kettering Cancer Center. To be clear, the title "doctor" or "Dr." does not necessarily imply medical qualifications. It is properly applied to any scholar who has earned a doctorate of philosophy (Ph.D.) in any field, including the humanities.

Nothing said in writing or in a conversation with Ralph W. Moss, Ph.D., or his coworkers, is medical advice or a substitute for qualified professional care. They are not qualified to prescribe for any medical condition and will not do so. Any recommendations are the personal opinions of lay people and are not in any sense prescriptions. If you have cancer, you should be under the care of appropriate medical professionals, including (but not necessarily limited to) oncologists.

You are encouraged to confirm the accuracy of the information included here or in any conversation, with other reliable sources. For instance, you are strongly encouraged to review this information with your healthcare professionals. As an aid to doing so, this text contains many scientific references that you can discuss with your physicians.

Neither Ralph W. Moss, Ph.D., nor his staff or coworkers, are liable for any indirect, consequential, special, exemplary, or other damages arising from the use of this text or in a conversation.

The responsibility is on you, the reader, to inform yourself about the beneficial and adverse effects of purported remedies, as well as harmful interactions with foods, supplements, or drugs. Text can only go so far in explaining reactions and interactions. The ultimate responsibility is on the reader to be a well-informed consumer.

Endometrial (Uterine) Cancer

Overview, Basics, and Key Statistics

This text describes the conventional understanding and treatment of endometrial cancer (EC, also called cancer of the uterus or cancer of the uterine body). The Moss Report will discuss the most important questions concerning endometrial cancer. There is also a separate section on (endometrial (uterine) sarcomas, which (if necessary) should be read in conjunction with the section on soft tissue sarcomas.

There are two primary parts of the uterus: the cervix (which is Latin for neck) and the upper rounded extremity, which is called the corpus or fundus of the uterus. Connecting the ovaries to the uterus are the Fallopian tubes, named after the early anatomist Gabriele Fallopio (1523-1562).

Female Reproductive System

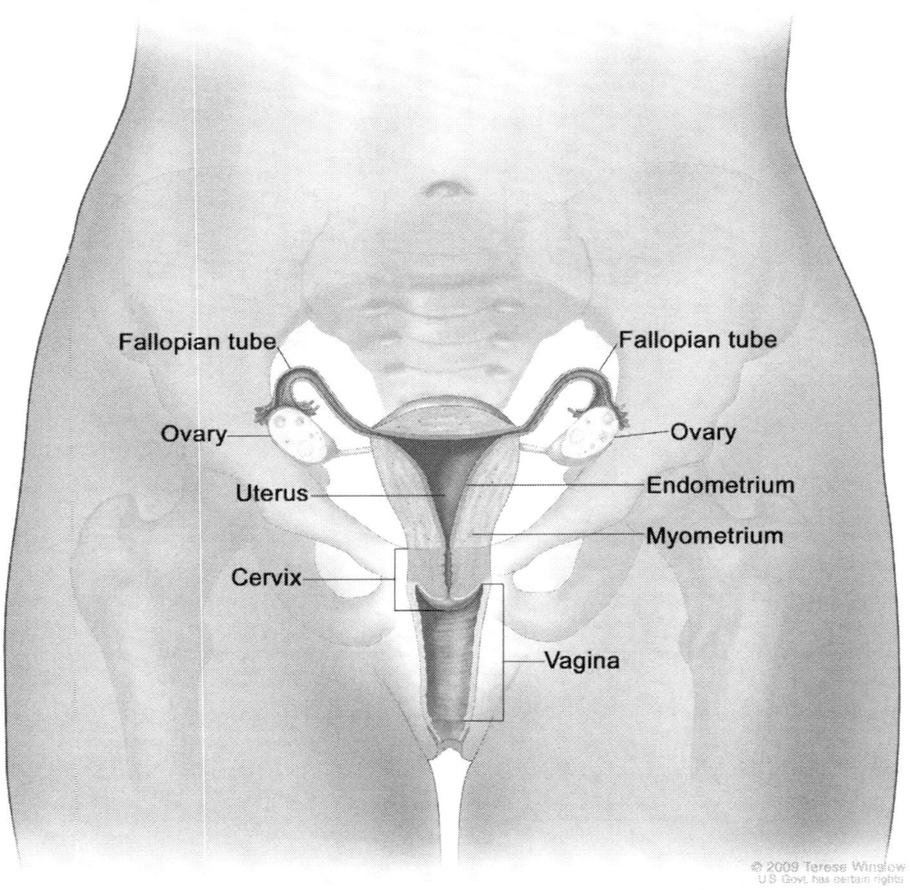

[Illustration courtesy of the National Cancer Institute.]

The endometrium is the mucous membrane that lines the uterine wall. Since it is in this lining that 90% of these cancers develop, most uterine cancers are also called "endometrial." When tumors occur in the muscular wall of the uterus or the myometrium, they are of a different cellular type called uterine sarcomas. They are much rarer than the endometrial type.

- (García-Martínez E, Egea Prefasi L, García-Donas J, et al. Current management of uterine sarcomas. Clin Transl Oncol. 2011;13:307-314; Older terms are "corpus carcinoma" and "fundic cancer")

There are an estimated 66,570 new cases of endometrial cancer in the U.S. each year. This represents 3.5% of all cancer cases. There are also an estimated 12,940 deaths, representing 2.1% of U.S. cancer deaths. The five-year relative survival is 81.1%. The trend for both occurrences and deaths is up slightly over the past few decades. By contrast, according to MSKCC, "uterine sarcoma is rare, making up less than 4% of all cancers of the uterus. Only 1,200 women are diagnosed with this disease in the United States each year."

According to the SEER Program of the NCI, the rate of new cases of uterine cancer was 28.1 per 100,000 women per year. The death rate was 4.9 per 100,000 women per year. Approximately 3.1% of women will be diagnosed with uterine cancer at some point during their lifetime. An estimated 813,861 women are living with uterine cancer in the United States.

History of Occurrence

The incidence of endometrial cancer has declined significantly over the last hundred or so years. Thus, in the 1880s, uterine cancer represented 30% of all cases of cancer. Even in 1940, it was the predominant form of cancer in women. The incidence continued to rise rapidly in the 1960s and the 1970s, primarily because of the increasing use of hormone replacement therapies (HRT). But it has been dropping steadily since the 1980s. Even with this decline, it is still the fourth most commonly diagnosed cancer in women in the U.S. Today, it is ten times less common than lung or breast cancer. The disease mostly affects postmenopausal women; the average age at diagnosis is 60 years.

- (American Cancer Society, Cancer Facts and Figures)

Figures

To visualize the impact of this disease on society, picture this:

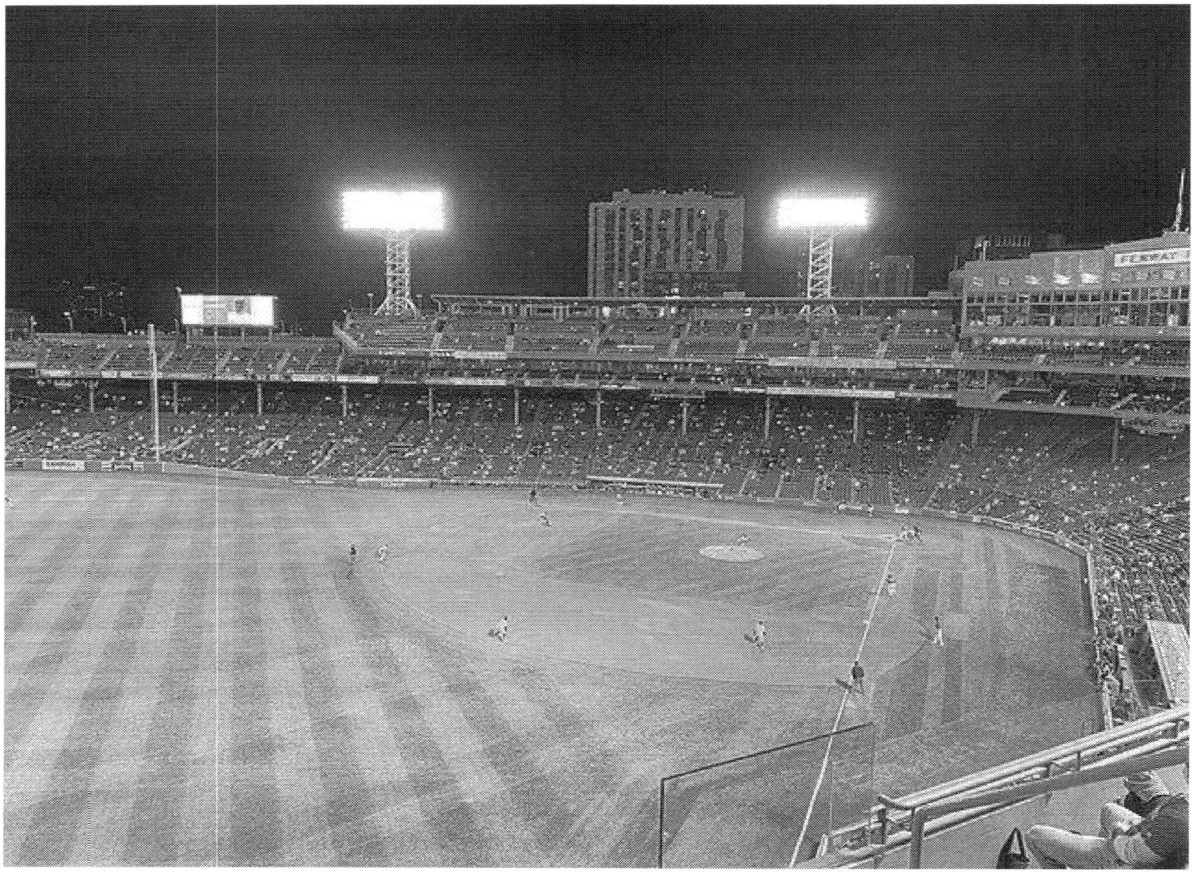

Fenway Park, Home of the Boston Red Sox (courtesy of Wikimedia Commons), 37,755 capacity

You could almost fill Fenway Park twice over with just one year's census of U.S. women newly diagnosed with endometrial cancer.

In this text, we are speaking about the most common tumor of the uterus, endometrial carcinoma. Toward the end of this section, we speak about certain rare tumors: carcinosarcomas, leiomyosarcomas, and other sarcomas affecting this organ.

Two Types of Endometrial Cancer

Perhaps the most important question is this: Which type of endometrial cancer are you concerned with? Endometrial cancers are broadly categorized as type I and type II tumors.

Type I tumors are dependent for their growth on the female hormone, estrogen; type II are independent of the effects of estrogen. Type I is more common (up to 80% of the whole) and tends to be discovered in younger women. These develop from a precursor lesion, called atypical hyperplasia. Their tumors are usually associated with an excess amount of estrogen. They also tend to be well differentiated and have minimal muscle invasion and, as a result, have a better outcome.

Type II, on the other hand, accounts for around 15% of tumors. They are found in an older population. About half of all relapses are said to occur among type II patients. Serous, clear-cell and grade 3 tumors occur primarily in this group. (Barakat 2013)

Causes and Prevention

Chronic exposure to the female hormone estrogen (unopposed by progesterone) is a risk factor for its development. Thus, late menopause, early menstruation, fewer pregnancies, long-term use of non-progestin-containing oral contraceptives, prolonged periods of non-ovulation, and the use of hormone replacement therapy (HRT) increase exposure to estrogen and therefore increase the risk of endometrial cancer.

Having previously had breast cancer is also a risk factor. Strangely, the long-term use of the anti-hormonal drug tamoxifen is linked to an increased incidence of endometrial cancer (primarily uterine sarcoma, an aggressive subtype) preceded by an initially non-cancerous condition (called hyperplasia) within the endometrium. Hyperplasia can become cancerous, accounting for the paradoxical link between tamoxifen and cancer driven by estrogen exposure.

About 1 in 500 women on tamoxifen following treatment for breast cancer develops endometrial cancer. For that reason, tamoxifen is usually not prescribed for more than five years. For postmenopausal women, there are now less dangerous alternatives—aromatase inhibitors such as letrozole (Femara®), anastrozole (Arimidex®), and exemestane (Aromasin®).

Obesity

Obesity is a major risk factor for endometrial cancer. The mechanism for this is unknown, but one possible mechanism is that adipocytes—or fat-storing cells—produce estrogen, thereby raising the body's own internally manufactured estrogen levels. (Sharma 2006; Kanasaki 2011; Libby 2014)

It has been estimated that approximately 80% of endometrial cancers occur in postmenopausal women who are overweight. Such cases are known as Type I endometrial cancer. Type II endometrial cancer occurs in women who are younger and typically not overweight. Such cancers are typically more aggressive than Type I tumors. (Carter 20006; Linkov 2014)

Previous irradiation for the treatment of cervical cancer is also associated with higher rates of subsequent endometrial cancer, and the cancers that arise as a result of this kind of previous radiation exposure tend to be of a more aggressive and even untreatable condition. (Kumar 2009; Elshaikh 2014)

Intentional Weight Loss

Intentional weight loss in postmenopausal women is associated with a lower risk of endometrial cancer. This is especially true among obese women, based on an analysis of the Women's Health Initiative (WHI) study. This observational study included data on weight loss among postmenopausal women. Compared to women who had stable weight, women with weight loss equal to or greater than 5% of their body weight had 29% less risk of endometrial cancer risk (HR = 0.71). This association was strongest among obese women with intentional weight loss (where the risk went down by 56%). The authors, including Rowan Chlebowski, MD, of UCLA wrote:

- “The results for endometrial cancer provide strong evidence supporting the hypothesis that intentional weight loss among obese postmenopausal women will lower their cancer risk.” (Luo 2017)

Lynch Syndrome

Women with Lynch syndrome, also known as hereditary non-polyposis colorectal cancer (HNPCC), also have an increased risk of endometrial cancer. In a study of 537 families with Lynch syndrome, the life-long risk for endometrial cancer by age 70 years is 54% for MLH1 mutation carriers, 21% for MSH2, and 16% for MSH6. But the estimated risk of endometrial cancer by age 40 years was no greater than 2%, regardless of the gene involved. (Bonadona 2011; de Pauw 2012; Hall 2016)

Do Soy and Soy Supplements Promote Endometrial Cancer?

This is a provocative question. A randomized trial (RCT) in Rome, published in 2004 in Fertility & Sterility, claimed that women who took soy phytoestrogen supplements—that is, estrogenic compounds derived from soy, which have been widely promoted as a safer method of easing the tribulations of menopause—were at higher risk of developing endometrial hyperplasia. (Under 2004)

However, a follow-up study in the U.S. found a reduced risk of endometrial cancer among those women taking phytoestrogens—but only among lean women. (Bandera 2009)

Other studies of phytoestrogens (from soy) have so far failed to confirm any harmful effects. (Ward 2010; Girardi 2014)

As you can imagine, the possible harmfulness of soy and soy-based supplements is a major concern in China, where people traditionally derive much of their protein from this ubiquitous plant. Looking at the issue of endometrial thickening (taken as a sign of developing cancer) a meta-analysis concluded:

- “A total of 23 trials were included in the current analysis. The overall results did not show a significant change of endometrial thickness after oral isoflavone supplementation.” (Liu 2016)

Reviewing this complicated picture, The Moss Report believes that both soy as a food source 9soy milk, tofu, etc.) and soy-based supplements are safe. However, most beans (including soy) do contain anti-enzyme compounds, such as trypsin inhibitors, which can lead to digestive problems. Protease inhibitors are proteins that form very stable complexes with digestive enzymes, “reducing their activity to very low levels.” (Savage 2003) If a person has digestive upset from intolerance to soy, they can always substitute nut milk for soymilk.

Detection and Diagnosis

The main symptom of endometrial cancer is a bloody discharge from the vagina. This is of course especially obvious in the post-menopausal woman, but it also may be mistaken for an extra-heavy period in pre- or peri-menopausal women.

Sentinel Node Biopsies

In the so-called SENTI-ENDO study, pelvic sentinel lymph nodes were detected in 89% of patients. The sensitivity of the test was 84% and its negative predictive value was 87%. (Ballester 2011)

Tumor Markers

Tumor markers are very useful in evaluating the success of treatment. Perhaps the most useful marker in endometrial cancer is the Cancer Antigen 125 Blood Test, also known as serum CA125 assay, which is more commonly associated with ovarian cancer than with endometrial cancer. However, it has been found that rising CA125 can also be predictive of recurrent endometrial cancer.

In one study of 214 endometrial cancer patients, CA125 was an independent risk factor for pelvic and para-aortic lymph node metastases. (Todo 2003)

It was also found that elevated levels of serum CA125 could also assist in predicting treatment response or in post-treatment surveillance. In the U.S. this test is currently available without a physician's involvement from Life Extension (via LabCorp and possibly Walgreens) for $61. (Patsner 1989)

HER2 for Endometrial Cancer? Probably Not.

Human epidermal growth factor receptor (HER2 or HER/2-neu) is only expressed in 8% of primary endometrial tumors and the HER2 expression was weak. (Leslie 2012)

In more aggressive subtypes of endometrial cancer, however, the presence of HER/2-neu overexpression presents the possibility of using the targeted agent trastuzumab (Herceptin®) to help control tumor growth. Research has been inconclusive, as this did not work in the phase II clinical trial. According to Gini F. Fleming of the University of Chicago:

- "Trastuzumab as a single agent did not demonstrate activity against endometrial carcinomas with HER2 overexpression or HER2 amplification...."(Fleming 2010; Pectasides 2007)

Grades of Tumor

While all endometrial carcinomas originate in the glands that line the uterus (and are therefore classified as adenocarcinomas), there are several subdivisions, by cell type and grade. Thus, about 90% of endometrial carcinomas are typical adenocarcinomas of the epithelial lining of the uterus. But the other 10% are rare kinds of uterine cancer such as clear cell carcinoma, papillary serous carcinoma, mucinous carcinoma, and papillary endometrial carcinoma. Generally speaking, these less common types of endometrial cancer affect older patients and are associated with earlier metastasis and a poorer prognosis.

Endometrial carcinomas are further divided by grade:

Grade 1

- Grade 1 is made up of well-differentiated cells that are still recognizable by their cell type. They have departed very little from normal cells and have the best prognosis.

Grade 2

- Grade 2 is made up of 50% or less poorly differentiated cells. These have an intermediary prognosis.

Grade 3

- Grade 3 tumors are then 50% poorly differentiated and have solid growth patterns. These have a worse prognosis.

Stages and Staging

[For a further explanation of stages and staging, please see Appendix C.]

What follows is a description of the treatment of each stage in greater detail.

Stage 0 Endometrial Hyperplasia

In endometrial hyperplasia, the lining of the uterus becomes thickened. This is essentially a benign condition but can lead to malignancy later on (about 10 to 30% of hyperplasia may ultimately develop into true cancers). If the condition is detected during screening, a woman may be advised to undergo a procedure known as dilation and curettage (D&C). (Gien 2008)

Stage I Endometrial Cancer

In stage Ia, the tumor is limited to just the endometrial lining of the uterus. The standard treatment is the surgical removal of the uterus, the Fallopian tubes, and the ovaries. The five-year survival rate after this procedure is between 90% to 95% and most patients are effectively cured.

For most stage Ia patients with endometrial cancer radiation are not required:

- "For patients with stage IA, grade 1 and 2 endometrioid adenocarcinoma (no or <50% myometrial invasion), adjuvant radiotherapy (RT) is not routinely recommended." (DeVita 2022: 1214)

In stage Ib, the tumor has invaded the uterine wall but is less than half of the wall's thickness. The treatment is the same as for stage Ia. However, in stage Ib, the surgeon will take a sample of the lymph nodes. No further treatment will be necessary if the tumor:

- Is either grade 1 or grade 2
- Involves the upper two-thirds of the uterus
- Has not invaded the blood vessels

- Has not invaded the uterus by more than one-third
- The abdominal (peritoneal cytology) washings show no malignant cells present,

However, if these conditions are not met, particularly if the tumor is grade 3, has invaded more than a third of the uterine wall, or has significantly invaded the blood vessels, then it is more likely to spread throughout the body. In such cases, external beam radiation is given. The usual dose to the pelvis and upper vagina after surgery is between 40 and 50 Grays (Gy), administered daily in divided doses, five days per week for four to five weeks.

Standard Treatments

Radiation Therapy

In stage Ic, the treatment is virtually the same as in stage I. Most gynecologists recommend whole pelvic radiation. But there is considerable disagreement over the role of adjuvant (i.e., postoperative) radiotherapy in the management of uterine cancers. (Creutzberg 2000)

Researchers have found that postoperative radiotherapy in stage I endometrial carcinoma reduces recurrence, but has no significant impact on overall survival (which is high in either case). Indeed, according to some studies, women who have not received radiation survive a recurrence better than those who receive radiation. They concluded:

- "Postoperative radiotherapy is not indicated in patients with stage I endometrial carcinoma below 60 years and patients with grade 2 tumors with superficial invasion" (Ibid.)

The choice of radiation or no radiation (and the type of radiation) is complicated. It often comes down to the risk factors for recurrence, impressions gained from inconclusive studies, and physician or patient preference. But it is hard for patients to express a rational preference when this issue is so technically complicated and there is relatively little data to support the choice of radiation.

In stage Ia, grade 3, and all stage II tumors the risk of recurrence is intermediate. Radiation will reduce the risk of local recurrence but there is no evidence that it prolongs overall survival. Vaginal cuff radiation (internal radiation of the upper part of the vagina) and pelvic radiation are said to be the preferred methods.

Stage II Endometrial Cancer

Stage II endometrial cancer used to be subdivided into stages IIa and IIb. However, since 2009, the Revised International Federation of Gynecology and Obstetrics Staging for Endometrial Cancer (FIGO) has dropped the subdivisions and dealt with all stage II endometrial cancers together. Stage II in essence means that the tumor has invaded the cervical stroma but has not extended beyond the uterus. (Pecorelli 2009)

The DeVita cancer textbook concludes that most data suggest that irradiation reduces the incidence of vaginal recurrence from 10% or 15% to less than 5% for patients with high-risk disease:

- "In summary, if postoperative radiation is needed in early-stage endometrioid adenocarcinoma, the preferred approach is intravaginal RT rather than pelvic RT in most cases." (Kaled 2022)

On the topic of preoperative radiotherapy for endometrial cancer, a different textbook states:

- "In patients with uterine [endometrial] cancer, preoperative irradiation has largely been abandoned in favor of postoperative irradiation, which can be planned when information from the surgical specimen is available and which avoids unnecessarily treating patients with the very-early-stage disease. Preoperative irradiation is sometimes used to treat patients with stage II endometrial cancer that grossly involves the cervix, and is used in some patients with bulky cervical cancers.' (Berek 2015)

Postoperative Radiation

Radiation will probably reduce the risk of recurrences. One prospective, randomized study compared patients who received one kind of radiotherapy (brachytherapy) with those who received two kinds (brachytherapy plus external beam irradiation). According to the DeVita textbook, the result was that there was no significant improvement in overall disease-specific survival. This study raised the possibility that patients whose disease was prevented from recurring at the local site "recurred instead at distant sites."

The DeVita authors have stated that other studies support the use of pelvic radiotherapy in patients with endometrioid or mucinous tumors. These need to be confined to the pelvis and suggest a high risk of recurrence to the pelvis.

Stage III Endometrial Cancer

In stage IIIa endometrial cancer, the uterine surface and/or the Fallopian tubes and ovaries are invaded by cancer, or malignant cells are present in the abdominal fluid, as detected through peritoneal washings (called 'lavage' or 'cytology'). Even popular books admit that after surgery, additional treatment is controversial and should be considered investigational. But most gynecological oncologists do recommend treatment with radiation therapy to the entire abdomen, as well as one of the following:

- Intra-abdominal radioactive substances, such as chromic phosphate;
- Hormonal treatment with progesterone; and/or
- Combination chemotherapy.

Stage IIIb is defined by the presence of metastases in the vagina. The standard treatment is abdominal hysterectomy, with the removal of the Fallopian tubes and ovaries on both sides, and, occasionally, the surgical excision of the metastases. This is followed by intensive radiotherapy.

Stage IIIc is defined by metastases to the pelvic and/or the para-aortic lymph nodes. Again, radiotherapy is generally used both pre-and-post-surgery. Many gynecologic oncologists also recommend adjuvant chemotherapy, such as cisplatin or carboplatin, doxorubicin (Adriamycin®), and/or cyclophosphamide (Cytoxan®), if the woman has positive aortic lymph node metastases.

Stage IV Endometrial Cancer

Stage IV endometrial cancer is defined by the presence of distant metastases, such as vital organs. Hormonal treatment with megestrol acetate (Megace®, a form of progesterone) is sometimes used as a palliative. The anti-hormonal drug tamoxifen is also used. Studies have shown that only about 20% of women respond positively to hormonal treatment, but these approaches are not considered curative.

Recurrent Endometrial Cancer

In recurrent diseases, hormonal therapy with progestogens (such as MPA), tamoxifen, or both has become standard. At one time, MPA was very widely used. However, it is now clear that beneficial outcomes are seen in only a minority of patients.

Chemo Drugs and Combinations

Scope of Chemotherapy: FDA-Approved Drugs

The U.S. Food and Drug Administration (FDA) has only approved one hormonal drug for endometrial cancer—megestrol acetate (Megace®). No chemotherapy drug has ever been explicitly approved for this disease. But many drugs have been, and are being used, in an off-label way and Medicare and other insurance plans generally will pay for such usage.

The National Comprehensive Cancer Network (NCCN) makes numerous recommendations for chemotherapy of advanced, metastatic, or recurrent endometrial cancer.

Single Drugs in Current Use

Here are the single drugs that the NCCN considers useful in endometrial cancer:

- Cisplatin
- Carboplatin
- Doxorubicin
- Doxorubicin, liposomal
- Paclitaxel
- Topotecan
- Bevacizumab
- Temsirolimus
- Docetaxel
- Ifosfamide (for carcinosarcoma)

Combinations in Current Use

[See Appendix G for Information on the National Comprehensive Cancer Network]

The NCCN recommendations also include combinations of the above agents. These regimens are preferred if the patient can tolerate the toxicity that is often associated with them. Most of them revolve around the use of three common drugs: doxorubicin, better known as Adriamycin®; one drug from the mineral platinum category; and/or one drug from the "taxane" category (originally derived from the Pacific Yew tree).

- Carboplatin + paclitaxel
- Cisplatin + doxorubicin
- Carboplatin + docetaxel
- Ifosfamide + paclitaxel
- Cisplatin + ifosfamide
- Cisplatin + doxorubicin + paclitaxel (This combination is rarely used because of its toxicity)

Surprisingly, the NCCN does not specify which of these numerous drugs or drug combinations is superior or desirable. The DeVita textbook has this to say about chemotherapy for stage IV, recurrent endometrial cancer:

- "Most women with recurrent or stage IV endometrial carcinoma should be assessed for treatment with cytotoxic chemotherapy. Current combination chemotherapy regimens can yield response rates of 50% to 60% with median OS [overall survival] about 12 to 15 months." (DeVita 2022)

In comparing clinical trials the key thing is their impact on the median overall survival (OS), the amount of time that the patient survives (not to be confused with progression-free survival, PFS). A second but no less important consideration is the side effects (a.k.a. adverse event) of the drug(s).

Results from different clinical trials can be difficult to compare, because some trials may recruit patients with more health challenges than other cherry-picked trials. That said, it is clear that the first trial to demonstrate a greater-than-one-year survival was that of Fleming (2004).

Most Effective Drug Combination

The best results in the history of endometrial cancer treatment were seen in the Miller (2012) trial, using the following: doxorubicin (Adriamycin®) + cisplatin + paclitaxel (Taxotere®) + G-CSF (granulocyte colony-stimulating factor, a kind of "rescue factor"). The response rate with this combination was over 50%, the progression-free survival (PFS) was 14 months, and the overall survival rate was 40.3 months. (Miller 2012)

This is extraordinary, considering that just 20 years before the median survival was typically 6 to 7 months. But one has to expect increased toxicity from this combination. (Thigpen 1994)

Trastuzumab + Chemotherapy

The standard treatment for women who have advanced or recurrent serous endometrial cancer is chemotherapy. However, new strategies are being tested for patients whose tumors overexpress human epidermal growth factor receptor 2 (HER2). In one randomized phase II trial with

61 such women, the addition of the anti-HER2 antibody Herceptin (trastuzumab) to chemotherapy improved the median progression-free survival (PFS) to 12.6 months vs. 8.0 months for chemotherapy alone. There was no reported increase in toxicity. (Fader 2018)

Because of this study, some oncologists now test for HER2 over-expression in advanced or recurrent endometrial serous carcinomas. They then may include trastuzumab with chemotherapy in the treatment protocol of such patients. But this remains an off-label indication and so might not be fully paid for by insurance. (One should check with one's insurance company in advance).

Targeted and Molecular Treatments

At this writing, there are 20 or so "molecular aberrations" associated with endometrial cancer. These consist of the loss, mutation, over-expression, or amplification of aberrant genes or gene products. Without listing all these, the reader can sense the enormous complexity of this evolving picture. One could spend the rest of this text explaining the complex web of connections between the various genetic components of the tumor—what someone once called a "tropical jungle" of mutations—and one still wouldn't get to the bottom of the problem.

Targeted Agents

Part of the complexity of this issue is to determine whether the patient in question has type I or type II endometrial cancer (see above discussion). These are two distinct subtypes of the disease, have different molecular signatures, and respond to different targeted drugs. When known, the text will indicate this fact in the discussion of targeted drugs.

While there are at present over 200 PubMed-indexed articles on "endometrial cancer" plus "targeted therapy," only a few of these present actual clinical trial data on this approach. The ones that exist are all phase II trials, in other words not randomized controlled trials (RCTs, which would by definition be phase III). It is axiomatic therefore that one needs to take their conclusions with a grain of salt.

Bevacizumab (Avastin®)

Bevacizumab (Avastin®) was the first of the anti-vascular growth factors. It is a monoclonal antibody, a kind of "guided missile" that targets a molecule called VEGF-A. The administration of the drug bevacizumab produced a response rate of 13.5% in patients who had had prior chemotherapy for endometrial cancer. Forty (40)% of the patients in a phase II trial were progression-free at six months. (Aghajanian 2011)

Cediranib

Cediranib (AZD 2171) is a potent medication currently under development. It targets at least three molecules associated with the abnormal growth of endometrial cancer. In a report, of 53 patients who had recurrent or persistent endometrial cancer, there was a partial response in 12.5%, and a six-month event-free survival in 29%. The median progression-free survival overall survival was 12.5 months. (Bender 2015)

Sunitinib (Sutent®)

There was a preliminary report at ASCO suggesting that sunitinib (Sutent®) produced a 15% response rate. (Correa 2010)

A later joint Canadian and California phase II clinical trial also showed promising results: It analyzed results in 33 women who received at least one dose of sunitinib and were included in the study. Six women (18.1%) had a partial response and six additional women (18.1%) had stable disease. A total of ten patients (30.3%) had disease control for at least 6 months and of these, seven were controlled for more than one year. The median progression-free survival (PFS) was 3 months, and the overall survival (OS) was 19.4 months. But side effects were frequent. Serious (grade 3) toxicity occurred in 30 patients and dose reductions were required in 52%. The most common serious toxicities were fatigue, hypertension, diarrhea, and low blood counts. The authors concluded:

- "Sunitinib therapy showed promising activity in women with recurrent endometrial cancer. Toxicity was seen frequently but was manageable. Anti-angiogenic agents warrant further investigation in EC to define which patients will derive the greatest benefit." (Castonguay 2014)

Temsirolimus (Torisel®)

There have been numerous studies of temsirolimus (Torisel®) as a second line of treatment for patients with endometrial cancer who had previously undergone chemotherapy but had recurrent disease. Many of these involve the administration of other agents as well as temsirolimus and are thus difficult to interpret.

There is a phase II study in which temsirolimus was given alone to women with recurrent or metastatic endometrial cancer. The patients were evaluated by whether or not they had had prior chemotherapy. In the "chemotherapy-naive group" 33 received four cycles of treatment. The Canadian authors said that 29 patients were evaluable for evaluation: four (or 14%) had a partial response and 20 (69%) had stable disease. In the chemotherapy-treated group, out of 25 evaluable patients, one (4%) had an independently confirmed partial response and 12 patients (48%) had stable disease. Strangely enough, molecular markers that were thought to be driving endometrial cancer "did not correlate with the clinical outcome." (Oza 2011)

Immunotherapy and Other Treatments

One big question is whether or not the new immune checkpoint blockade (ICB) can be used successfully in endometrial cancer. The preliminary answer is, Yes. Studies of biopsy samples of endometrial patients show that the levels of PD-1 (on immune cells) and PD-L1 (on cancer cells) are higher than in either ovarian or cervical cancer. In one study, PD-L1 was found in 67% to 100% of samples. The presence of PD-L1 is usually taken as a sign that the patient has a better chance of responding to immune checkpoint inhibitors, in particular the drugs nivolumab (Opdivo®) and pembrolizumab (Keytruda®).

One issue being explored is whether or not the presence or absence of "mismatch repair" (MMR) genes affect one's response to these new drugs. There has been a phase 2 trial of pembrolizumab to explore this question. Although mainly a study of colorectal cancer, there were a few endometrial cancer patients in the trial who were MMR-deficient, and indeed they had a higher rate of progression-free survival (PFS) than patients with MMR-proficient tumors.

The conclusion of gynecologic oncologists at the University of California, Irvine (UCI) Medical Center was as follows:

- "Existing evidence suggests that endometrial cancer is sufficiently immunogenic to be a reasonable candidate for active and/or passive immunotherapy....Immune checkpoint inhibitors may be used effectively in the treatment of MMR-deficient endometrial cancers, and trials exploring this hypothesis are currently in development." (Longoria 2015)

People whose cancer cells have a lot of "mismatch repair" (MMR) capacity are less likely to derive benefits from ICB. But MMR-deficient examples of colon cancer are particularly susceptible to immune checkpoint blockade. There have been several clinical reports that this is the case.

For example, there was a phase II study of the drug pembrolizumab (Keytruda®) given to patients with MMR-deficient tumors. All patients had been heavily pretreated with chemotherapy. The results were presented at a meeting of the American Society of Clinical Oncology (ASCO). Patients with MMR-deficient colon cancer had a 50% objective response rate (ORR) and 89% disease control rate (either objective response or stable disease).

By contrast, the ORR was 0% and the disease control rate was just 16% in the patients with MMR-proficient colon cancer. After six months, none of the MMR-deficient patients had progressed (i.e., had a recurrence), but patients in the MMR-proficient group were doing very poorly. (Le 2016; Le 2017)

In the CheckMate 142 trial, MMR-deficient patients received a competing immune checkpoint drug, nivolumab (Opdivo®). In another preliminary report at the 2016 annual meeting of ASCO, this new form of immunotherapy benefited those with MMR-deficient tumors but not those with MMR-proficient tumors. However, one should bear in mind that most colon cancers are MMR proficient.

There is also evidence that combining ICB with two drugs, such as cobimetinib plus atezolizumab might make ICB effective even in MMR-proficient tumors. (Overman 2016)

Pembrolizumab and lenvatinib in advanced endometrial cancer

There was a randomized trial that evaluated the immune checkpoint drug pembrolizumab (Keytruda®) and lenvatinib (Lenvima®), a kinase inhibitor, versus just chemotherapy (either doxorubicin or paclitaxel, based on the physician's choice). There were over 800 patients in the trial who had advanced endometrial cancer that had progressed on platinum-based chemotherapy. The combination of pembrolizumab and lenvatinib improved overall survival (OS) by 18.3 months versus 11.4 months for the chemo, for an absolute gain of 6.9 months. Among those who had MMR-proficient tumors (supposedly not susceptible to immune checkpoint inhibitors) the improvement for an absolute gain of 5.4 months. This was a significant finding that got little attention. MMR proficiency is often said to disqualify patients from receiving immunotherapy. However, here it did not seem to make much of a difference. Of course, in a trial of this design, it is impossible to say how much of the improvement was due to the checkpoint inhibitor (pembrolizumab) and how much was due to the multiple kinase inhibitor, lenvatinib.

According to the UpToDate authors:

- "Pembrolizumab plus lenvatinib is an appropriate option for patients with advanced, platinum-resistant endometrial cancer that is proficient in MMR, although we continue to suggest immunotherapy alone for such cancers that are MMR-deficient, based on previous data."

Immune Checkpoint Inhibitors Plus Chemotherapy In Advanced Endometrial Cancer (2023)

For people with advanced endometrial cancer (a type of uterus cancer), there's a common treatment using two drugs: carboplatin and paclitaxel. However, new studies are looking at adding another type of drug to the mix, called immune checkpoint inhibitors (or ICIs for short), to see if they can make the treatment even better.

Two recent studies found that when adding either of the ICIs, named dostarlimab or pembrolizumab, to the usual drug combo, patients' cancer took longer to get worse. Specifically, those who added dostarlimab also had a better chance of living longer. This was most notable in a group of patients whose cancer had a specific trait called mismatch repair deficiency (dMMR). In this group, 83% of those treated with dostarlimab were still alive at the 24-month mark, compared to 59% without it. (Eskander 2023; Mirza 2023)

So, for those with advanced endometrial cancer and the dMMR trait, doctors are now suggesting adding either dostarlimab or pembrolizumab to the usual treatment.

Dostarlimab in Advanced, Platinum-Refractory Endometrial Cancer

In a single-arm study that included 70 or so patients with advanced endometrial cancer, the objective response rate to the immune checkpoint inhibitor dostarlimab (Jemperli®) was 42%. Of the total patient population, 13% experienced a complete response. (Oaknin 2020)

The most common serious to severe side effects were anemia, colitis, and diarrhea. But each of these occurred in fewer than 5% of the patient population. These results supported the U.S. Food and Drug Administration's (FDA) approval of dostarlimab (Jemperli®) for patients with advanced or recurrent dMMR endometrial cancer that has progressed on prior platinum-based chemotherapy.

Progestin Therapy of Early-Stage Endometrial Cancer

Endometrial carcinoma can be treated with progestins rather than a hysterectomy in women who have the lowest stage of the disease and who plan future pregnancies. In the largest study yet to compare outcomes after progestin therapy vs. surgery, women with stage IA disease had similar five-year survival with either treatment (98%), whereas progestin therapy was associated with lower five-year survival in women with stage IB disease (approximately 75 versus 98%).

According to Gini Fleming, MD of the University of Chicago Medical Center and Paul A DiSilvestro, MD of the Alpert School of Medicine at Brown University, fertility-preserving treatment of endometrial carcinoma is considered reasonable in appropriately selected women with stage

IA disease, but use in higher-stage disease appears to compromise survival. (Ruiz 2017)

Uterine Papillary Serous Carcinoma (UPSC)

As stated, about 90% of uterine tumors are of the adenocarcinoma type. (An adenocarcinoma is a tumor that arises in a surface layer of cells, containing glandular elements.) But the remaining 10% are of rarer types: papillary serous carcinoma is one such. (Other rare kinds are clear cell carcinomas and mucinous carcinomas.) Papillary serous carcinomas of the uterus are usually referred to in the literature as uterine papillary serous carcinoma, abbreviated UPSC.

[NOTE: This type of cancer can be confused with the papillary villoglandular subtype of endometrioid adenocarcinoma, which carries a significantly better prognosis. Patients given this diagnosis should make sure that their slides have been reviewed by an outstanding pathology department. If you have any doubts about this score, have them sent to a major academic pathology department, such as Memorial Sloan-Kettering Cancer Center in New York City.]

Approximately 3,500 new diagnoses of UPSC are made each year in the U.S. UPSC was named by analogy with a different tumor, papillary serous carcinoma of the ovaries or fallopian tubes. Papillary means shaped like a nipple—referring to the way these tumors tend to grow. The term "serous" refers to a tumor that produces a serum or a substance that has a watery consistency. A serous, or mucous, discharge was among the earliest found symptoms of endometrial cancers. Their detection generally preceded the more common tumors that are first detected from erosions of the uterus wall.

Uterine cancers were originally sub-classified by various cell types. Almost all endometrial cancers arise from glands in the lining of the uterus. If an endometrial carcinoma also contained a component of malignant squamous cells it was—logically enough—classified as adenosquamous carcinoma. These adenosquamous carcinomas account for most of the remaining cases. There is also a rare uterine sarcoma. Finally, a small number of women are found to have clear cell carcinomas of the uterus. Or at least that was where things stood a while back.

Then, Michael Hendrickson, MD, of Stanford University Medical School, Palo Alto, described another type of adenocarcinoma, whose appearance was strikingly similar to papillary serous carcinoma. This type of uterine cancer is now recognized as a subtype in the World Health Organization (WHO) Histologic Classifications of Endometrial Cancer. (Hendrickson 1982; Gunderson 2006:909)

Under the microscope, a serous tumor is characterized by papillary (nipple-like) projections, lined by bizarre cells with scanty cytoplasm, and it appears to detach easily. Microscopic structures called Psammoma bodies and clear cell features are also frequently seen. (Murphy 1995)

Hendrickson and colleagues reviewed 256 cases of stage I uterine adenocarcinoma treated at Stanford University Hospital in California and found 26 cases of uterine papillary serous carcinoma (UPSC). They described this entity as a clinically aggressive and microscopically distinct form of adenocarcinoma, which closely resembles ovarian papillary serous carcinoma. Thus, 10% of the cases were classified as UPSC—a surprisingly high number for a previously unknown kind of cancer.

Biologically, these cancers behave similarly to clear cell cancers. They tend to metastasize readily, often via the peritoneal route. Spread beyond the uterus is found upon exploratory laparotomy in more than half of the patients who are believed to have stage I disease.

These lesions are easily recognized through microscopic examination. They typically feature a high degree of “anaplasia” (disorganization) in the cells as well as a papillary growth pattern. Invasion of the lymph channels is a frequent finding as well. They tend to be poorly differentiated and are highly associated with invasion of the outer half of the myometrium (muscular uterine wall) as well as with extra-uterine spread.

As with most cancers, the degree of tumor differentiation is a strong predictor of survival outcome, with the worst outcomes associated with the least differentiated tumors.

In studies, what has made UPSC distinctive is the fact that the relapse rate among patients who have stage I UPSC is around 50%, which is five times the rate that one would expect with the more ordinary forms of endometrial cancer.

Patients with stage 1 UPSC have also been found to do significantly worse than a similar group of non-papillary stage 2 or even stage 3 adenocarcinoma patients. Forty percent of the patients with stage I UPSC patients have a deep invasion of the myometrium, as compared with 12% of those who have the other types of adenocarcinoma.

Women with UPSC deeply invading the myometrium also tend to fare worse than those with deeply invasive lesions of the more usual types of uterine cancer. This is reflected in the relapse rates (after surgery alone) of 63% for UPSC compared to just 30% in those with “ordinary” endometrial cancers.

Put another way, of the stage I patients whose initial site of failure was in the upper abdomen, almost all had UPSC. Thus, the Stanford authors concluded, UPSC shares the tendency of its ovarian counterpart to spread over and into the peritoneal surfaces.

In addition to their original study of stage I patients, they also followed the cases of 26 other patients who had more advanced stages of UPSC. Of these, only four survived.

Eleven of these women developed what is called “abdominal carcinomatosis,” which is the spread of cancer diffusely throughout the abdomen. The researchers, therefore, concluded that UPSC is a clinically aggressive cancer that should be distinguished from other types of primary cancer of the uterus.

In cases of invasive UPSC, the method of spread is similar to that of ovarian surface epithelial carcinomas. The treatment implication was that UPSC patients, even more than other endometrial cancer patients, require aggressive adjuvant treatment after surgery. The conventional options include upper abdominal and pelvic irradiation and/or chemotherapy, even when such patients first present with ostensible stage I disease. (Hendrickson 1982; Rauh-Hain 2010)

After their initial report on 26 patients, the Stanford authors reported on an additional 10 patients. Upon operation, half of these patients (5/10) who seemed to have stage I disease turned out to have more advanced disease. Most were treated aggressively. The use of preoperative intracavitary radiation was not found to be of value. (Eifel 1983)

Adjuvant postoperative radiation was administered to the abdomen and pelvis in six patients, of whom four remained free of disease within the treated area. Two patients received adjunctive hormonal treatment and chemotherapy, and neither of these patients suffered recurrences. Two patients received no adjunctive therapy. One of these patients suffered recurrence initially in the vagina with subsequent recurrence in the lungs and lymph nodes above the collar bone. These findings are suggestive (but not conclusive) of the value of conventional adjunctive (additive) therapy. (Ibid.)

Because of the rarity of this subtype of endometrial cancer, there have not been very many studies of the disease. Most of the literature consists of retrospective reviews from single institutions of all the patients with this disease that passed through their doors over a specified period. These studies are informative, to be sure, but they are not as useful in decision-making as randomized controlled trials (RCTs). (Black 2016)

One review put their UPSC findings this way:

- "In the setting of optimally debulked advanced-stage disease, a combination of radiation and chemotherapy may be indicated. In the setting of recurrent or suboptimally debulked advanced disease, a platinum-based regimen is recommended. Although comprising a minority of the women with endometrial cancer, women with UPSC do account for a disproportionate number of the recurrences." (Gehrig 2007; Kawano 2011)

[NOTE: A "platinum-based regimen" means the obligatory inclusion of either the anticancer drug cisplatin or carboplatin or more rarely oxaliplatin.]

UPDATE 1: Pelvic Intensity Modulated Radiation therapy in GYN Cancers

Intensity-modulated radiation therapy (IMRT) is a form of radiation that changes the intensity of the radiation in different parts of a single radiation beam. In a trial involving 289 patients with endometrial or cervical cancer receiving radiation to the pelvis, patients receiving IMRT had less high-level diarrhea compared with conventional radiation therapy (6%).

After three years, patients in the IMRT group had improvements in urinary function, while those in the conventional radiation arm had a decline in function. These results support the use of IMRT in gynecologic malignancies. (Yeung 2022)

Uterine (Endometrial) Sarcomas

The discussion of endometrial cancer generally focuses on carcinomas, which represent between 93% and 97% of all uterine cancers. These relatively rare sarcomas are further classified as follows:

- Endometrial stromal tumors
- Smooth muscle tumors
- Miscellaneous mesenchymal tumors

In the mixed epithelial and mesenchymal tumors category, the World Health Organization (WHO) includes the following:

- Adenosarcomas
- Carcinosarcomas, a.k.a. malignant mixed Müllerian tumors (MMT)

Carcinosarcoma

Although numerically small, uterine carcinosarcoma (also referred to as mixed Müllerian tumor) accounts for ~15% of uterine cancer-associated deaths in the U.S. This disease is more commonly found in African-American women. The prolonged use of the anti-breast cancer drug tamoxifen is also a risk factor. Among women who were treated with tamoxifen for breast cancer, the relative risk of developing uterine carcinosarcoma was found to be 4.62 (i.e., they had more than 4x the chance of getting the disease than the general population). Previous radiation therapy to the pelvis is another risk factor. It is rare in women under 50 but the incidence rises sharply after the age of 50.

According to the DeVita cancer textbook,

- "Uterine carcinosarcomas are aggressive tumors with a generally poor prognosis; 5-year OS [overall survival, ed.] has been reported to be about 30%, and for those with stage I disease it is about 50%." (Alektiar 2022)

Radiation Therapy for Carcinosarcoma

Adjuvant radiotherapy is often used for early-stage uterine carcinosarcoma. There was a European clinical trial that addressed the question of postoperative pelvic RT in stage I-II uterine sarcomas. A total of 224 patients underwent total abdominal hysterectomy with bilateral salpingo-oophorectomy (TAHBSO). This is the surgical removal of the entire uterus, the ovaries, the fallopian tubes, and the cervix. In this group, there were 103 leiomyosarcomas, 91 carcinosarcomas, and 28 endometrial stromal sarcomas.

The 5-year local-regional recurrence rate was 18.8% in the pelvic RT arm compared to 35.9% in the surgery-alone arm.

Oddly, the five-year cumulative incidence of distant relapse was 45.3% for the pelvic RT versus 33.6% for surgery alone, but the difference was not statistically significant. There was no significant difference in progression-free survival (PFS) or overall survival (OS) between the two arms.

Chemotherapy for Uterine Carcinosarcoma

The DeVita authors summarize the situation:

- "There are few randomized trials of adjuvant chemotherapy in early-stage carcinosarcoma, and results of small single institution series are difficult to interpret, although platinum-based therapy generally appears to be of benefit." (Ibid.)

The only drugs that have shown clear-cut activity in carcinosarcoma are:

- Cisplatin
- Doxorubicin
- Ifosfamide

These are non-curative and also tend to have considerable toxicity. Ifosfamide's side effects include a reduction in white blood cells (granulocytopenia) and central nervous system (CNS) toxicity.

Combinations of chemotherapy do produce higher response rates (i.e., tumor shrinkages) but the median survival is generally not improved over single agents and is generally under 1 year. To my knowledge, the longest response was a median overall survival (OS) of 26 months, using the three-drug combination of cisplatin + doxorubicin + ifosfamide. (van Rijswijk 2003)

Targeted or antiangiogenic agents do not seem to be at all effective in carcinosarcomas of the uterus.

Leiomyosarcoma

Leiomyosarcomas are the most common uterine sarcomas. Because they generally cause either abnormal bleeding or a pelvic mass, they are usually diagnosed in stage I. About 0.5% of women undergoing hysterectomy for benign conditions will be found to have leiomyosarcoma.

Surgery for Leiomyosarcoma

The standard surgical treatment for stage I disease is a simple hysterectomy with bilateral salpingo-oophorectomy (BSO). Lymph node involvement is rare at this stage and so lymph node dissection is generally not required.

But chest imaging is important since 10% of patients do have lung metastases at the time of diagnosis. Five-year survival for stage I is 50 to 60%, and for stage II it is about 25%.

Radiation for Leiomyosarcoma

So far at least adjunctive radiation therapy has produced no improvement in either local control or survival in leiomyosarcoma. (Reed 2008)

Chemotherapy for Leiomyosarcoma

There is only a small amount of data on the chemotherapy of leiomyosarcoma. The Gynecological Oncology Group (GOG) performed a small study of doxorubicin (Adriamycin®) after tumor resection. Stage I or II leiomyosarcomas and carcinosarcomas were included. Of 25 patients with leiomyosarcoma in the doxorubicin group, 11 (44%) recurred, compared with 14 (61%) in the observation group. (Omura 1985)

The French Sarcoma Group conducted a trial of adjuvant chemotherapy with doxorubicin, ifosfamide, and cisplatin followed by RT versus RT alone in patients who had localized uterine sarcomas. The three-year disease-free survival (DFS) was 55% in patients who received chemo-radiation versus 41% for RT alone. The three-year overall survival rates were 81% versus 69%, respectively. (Pautier 2013)

Pazopanib (Votrient®) for Leiomyosarcoma

Pazopanib hydrochloride (Votrient®) is one of the rare drugs that was approved (in 2012) by the U.S. Food and Drug Administration (FDA) for the treatment of soft tissue sarcomas. It is taken in tablet form for patients who had previously received chemotherapy. The approval was based on a trial of 369 patients who received either pazopanib or a placebo. Forty-three% of the patients had leiomyosarcomas. The median progression-free survival (PFS) was 4.6 months with pazopanib versus 1.6 months with a placebo. The objective response rate (RR) was 4% for pazopanib versus 0% for placebo. The median overall survival (OS) was 12.6 months for pazopanib versus 10.7 months for placebo, for a gain of 1.9 months. According to the FDA Website, common side effects included fatigue, diarrhea, nausea, weight loss, hypertension, decreased appetite, vomiting, tumor pain, hair color changes, musculoskeletal pain, headache, dyspnea, and skin hypo-pigmentation. Less common side effects were liver toxicity, arterial and venous thrombotic events, hemorrhage, gastrointestinal perforation, fistula formation, pneumothorax, and left ventricular dysfunction.

Regorafenib for Leiomyosarcoma

There was a randomized trial of the new drug regorafenib (Stivarga®) versus placebo in leiomyosarcoma and other types of soft tissue sarcoma. The 6-month overall survival rate of the LMS patients was 87.0% versus 75.9% with placebo, for a gain of 11.1%. The median progression-free survival (PFS) of LMS patients was 4.0 months with regorafenib (RE) versus 1.9 months with placebo, for an absolute gain of 2.1 months. The median PFS of other sarcoma patients was 4.6 months with regorafenib versus 1.0 months with placebo, for a gain of 3.6 months. Olivier Mir of the Gustave Roussy Cancer Institute, Paris, concluded that regorafenib "demonstrates promising activity and an acceptable toxicity profile that warrants further clinical evaluation in LMS" and other types of sarcoma patients. (Mir 2015)

Endometrial stromal sarcomas are very rare tumors. They comprise 0.2% of all uterine malignancies and 6 to 20% of uterine sarcomas. Since there are ~60,000 new cases of the uterine corpus in the U.S. each year, we can infer that there are about 120 such cases of endometrial stromal cancer in the U.S. each year (out of a female population of 163,000,000+). Thus, the odds of getting such cancer are less than one in a million.

In most cases, the disease is diagnosed early. The primary treatment is a hysterectomy (surgery). Lymph node dissection does not increase survival. Removal of the ovaries is generally recommended, but recent studies have not found that this impacts survival. A very small series of patients have suggested that radiation therapy decreases the relapse rate. However, a retrospective review found a nearly identical "cure" rate with or without postoperative radiation. Adjuvant hormonal therapy is often recommended, although there is no prospective data to justify its use. The role of chemotherapy is "unclear'' (DeVita). In advanced disease, various combinations of gemcitabine + docetaxel, doxorubicin, and ifosfamide have shown some short-lived responses. (Tanner 2012)

APPENDICES

The full set of *Treatment Guide* Appendices is available at the link below.

https://www.themossreport.com/appendices.pdf

APPENDIX A: FURTHER SOURCES OF INFORMATION

This full list of resources is kept up to date and is available at:

https://www.themossreport.com/appendices.pdf

Find the Best in Integrative Oncology at *The Moss Report*

Your path to understanding and managing cancer doesn't end here. We invite you to visit our comprehensive resource: *The Moss Report*. Our website offers an extensive information on a wide range of integrative oncology topics, designed to empower you with knowledge and choices in your cancer treatment journey. We help you answer these critical questions:

Where Should I Go?

Find out, in our *Doctors and Clinics* section, and our *Practitioner Map*

Clinic Overviews: Uncover detailed information about clinics specializing in cancer treatment across Mexico, Europe, the United States, and other parts of the world.

Unique Video Content: Explore our in-depth series – *Cancer Clinic Tours*.

This section of our website offers an in-person perspective on visits to dozens of integrative oncology clinics around the world. The videos feature Dr. Moss's probing interviews with the clinics' medical directors, providing in-depth insights into their treatment methodologies and a clear understanding of their philosophy and approach to cancer treatment. This comprehensive look at integrative oncology clinics is available exclusively at www.themossreport.com.

The Moss Report Integrative Oncology Practitioner Map features over 2000 resources and is unique to www.themossreport.com.

What Foods Should I Eat and Which Supplements Should I Take?

The Moss Method: Fight Cancer Naturally

The companion book to this *Guide*, is Dr. Moss' magnum opus, with the summation of over 50 years of research into less-toxic, more natural approaches to fighting cancer.

Focus on Diet and Natural Therapies: *The Moss Method™* emphasizes the power of a Mediterranean diet and natural therapies in the fight against cancer, providing a holistic perspective on healing.

APPENDIX C: STAGES AND STAGING

This appendix discusses the question of how one "stages" cancer. The words "staging" and "staging system" has a special meaning when it comes to cancer. According to the *NCI Cancer Dictionary,* staging means:

- "Performing exams and tests to learn the extent of cancer within the body, especially whether the disease has spread from where it first formed to other parts of the body. It is important to know the stage of the disease to plan the best treatment."

A "staging system" means:

- "A system that is used to describe the extent of cancer in the body. Staging is usually based on the size of the tumor and whether cancer has spread from where it started to nearby areas, lymph nodes, or other parts of the body."

Staging is of vital importance in making treatment decisions for any particular cancer. As the American Cancer Society website puts it:

- "For most types of cancer, doctors need to know how much cancer there is and where it is (among other things) to help determine the best treatment options. For example, the best treatment for early-stage cancer may be surgery or radiation, while a more advanced-stage cancer may need treatments that reach all parts of the body, such as chemotherapy, targeted drug therapy, or immunotherapy."

Staging is an attempt to discover the true extent of cancer in the human body. To do so, physicians look at the primary, or main, tumor. What are its size and location and has it grown into other nearby areas? They look for affected lymph nodes. Finally, they look to see if cancer has spread to other organs, including ones distant from the original primary site.

The stage of cancer is typically a composite of three figures. For a long time, physicians relied upon the so-called Jewett-Strong-Marshall system, which measured the depth of invasion of the tumor. But today almost everyone uses the universal TNM system. This gives a more detailed picture of the local, regional, and general status of the disease.

The TNM System

The TNM system is an almost universally adopted method of classifying solid tumors by reference to three key characteristics. These are the size and extent of the tumors (the "T" in TNM), the spread of cancer to the lymph nodes ("N"), and the extent of non-local metastases ("M").

There are of course different systems that are used to stage cancer. The most common and useful one for most types of cancer is the TNM system. Two organizations, the American Joint Committee on Cancer (AJCC) and the Union for International Cancer Control (UICC), maintain this TNM classification system to help doctors stage many different types of cancer-based on common standards.

In this system, the stage is determined AFTER the cancer has been assigned a letter or number to describe the key features of cancer.

- **T** describes the original (primary) **tumor**.
- **N** tells whether cancer has spread to the nearby lymph **nodes**.
- **M** tells whether cancer has spread (**metastasized**) to distant parts of the body

The TNM score yields crucial information that helps assign a particular cancer to its current **stage.** This is a process of determining the degree to which any particular cancer has grown or spread. Typically, doctors assign a Roman numeral from I to IV to any solid cancer. The letter "I" refers to an isolated tumor, while IV is cancer that has spread distantly (or is at its greatest extent).

Here is a good description of the various TNM categories (from the ACS website):

[Beginning of quotation from the ACS website:]

The primary tumor (T category)

"The **T category** can be assigned a letter or a number:

- **TX** means there's no information about the primary tumor, or it can't be measured.
- **T0** means there is no evidence of a primary tumor (it cannot be found).
- **Tis** means that the cancer cells are only growing in the layer of cells where they started, without growing into deeper layers. This may also be called **in situ** cancer or **pre-cancer**.
- A number after the T (such as **T1, T2, T3, or T4**) might describe the tumor size and/or amount of spread into nearby structures. The higher the T number, the larger the tumor and/or the more it has grown into nearby tissues.

The lymph nodes (N category)

Lymph nodes near the primary tumor are usually checked to find out if cancer has spread into them. Lymph nodes are small, bean-shaped collections of immune cells. Many types of cancer often spread to nearby lymph nodes before they reach other parts of the body.

The **N category** can be assigned a letter or a number:

- **NX** means there's no information about the nearby lymph nodes, or they can't be assessed.
- **N0** means nearby lymph nodes do not contain cancer.
- A number after the N (such as **N1, N2, or N3**) might describe the size, location, and/or the number of nearby lymph nodes affected by cancer. The higher the N number, the greater the cancer spread to nearby lymph nodes.

Metastasis (M category)

Doctors might also look at other parts of the body to see if cancer has spread. The cancer spread to parts of the body far from the primary tumor is known as **metastasis**.

The **M category** is assigned a number:

- **M0** means that no distant cancer spread has been found.
- **M1** means that cancer has been found to have spread to distant organs or tissues.

[End of quotation from ACS]

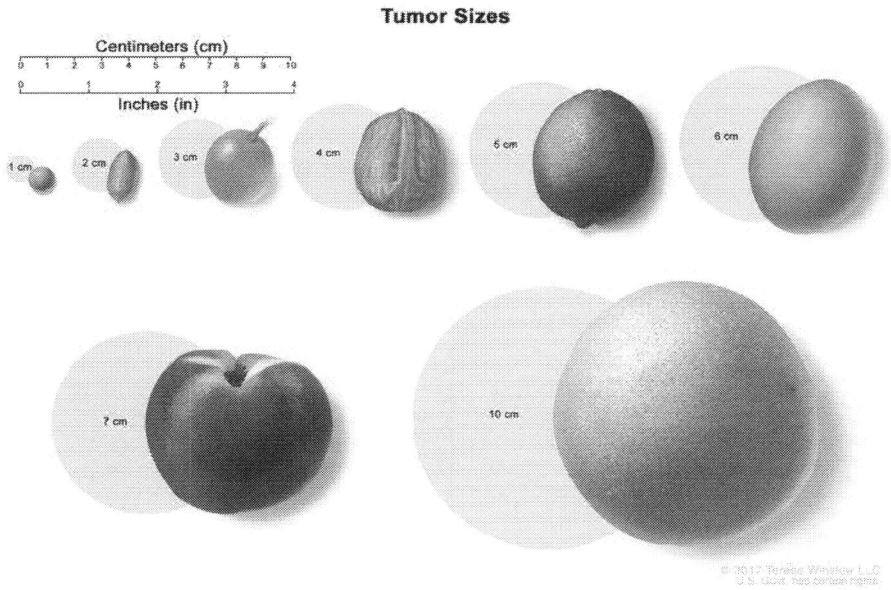

•

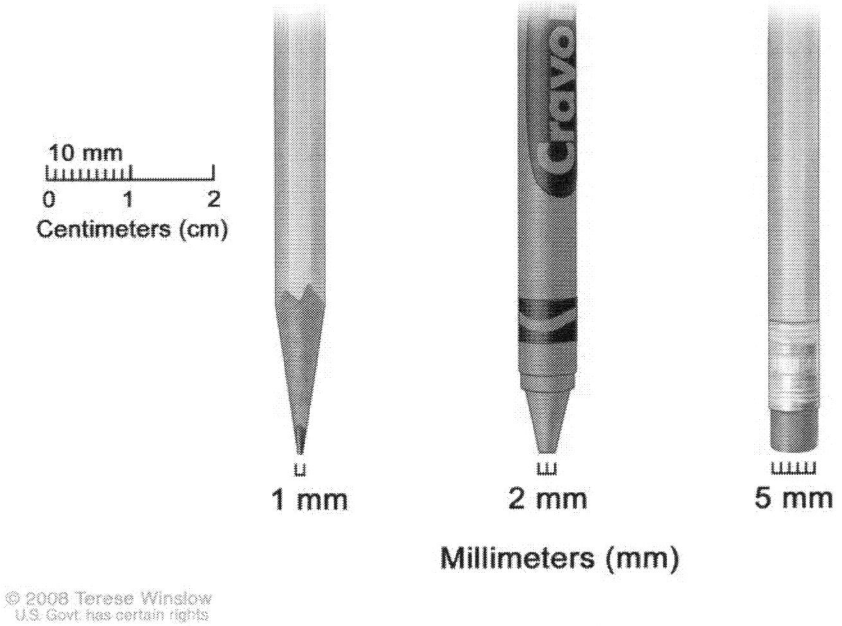

•

[These illustrations and the descriptions of stages are courtesy of the National Cancer Institute website, www.cancer.gov]

Appendix G: The National Comprehensive Cancer Network (NCCN)

Needless to say, we cannot go through all of the National Comprehensive Cancer Network (NCCN) recommendations, but we will touch on some of the most important ones.

The National Comprehensive Cancer Network (www.nccn.org) is an alliance of U.S. cancer centers. Their writing and review panels are made up of experts who diagnose and treat all cancers, but with a focus on complex, aggressive, or uncommon cancers.

The National Comprehensive Cancer Network (nccn.org) is an alliance of U.S. cancer centers. Their experts diagnose and treat all cancers, but with a focus on complex, aggressive, or uncommon cancers. They more or less set the standard for doctors and hospitals in the U.S. and abroad. The NCCN gives the categories of evidence and consensus for all treatments. That way readers can judge the strength of the particular recommendation:

> Category 1: Based upon high-level evidence, there is uniform NCCN consensus that the intervention is appropriate.
> Category 2A: Based upon lower-level evidence, there is uniform NCCN consensus that the intervention is appropriate.
> Category 2B: Based upon lower-level evidence, there is NCCN consensus that the intervention is appropriate.
> Category 3: Based upon any level of evidence, there is major NCCN disagreement that the intervention is appropriate.
> All recommendations are category 2, unless otherwise stated.

Needless to say, we cannot go through all of the NCCN's detailed algorithms and recommendations, but will only touch on some of the most important ones. NCCN has numerous and detailed charts for every stage of almost every kind of cancer. We will focus on the areas of greatest interest to our readers. These are the particular drugs and drug combinations that are recommended as a systemic treatment for each stage, and in particular, those that have NCCN's category 1 or at least 2A recommendations.

The NCCN recommendations are thorough and complete. Yet they also are so detailed that they can become difficult to interpret and understand. This is a text meant essentially for patients, thus, we will not try to give a detailed description. Interested readers can and should consult the freely available NCCN guidelines for him or herself.

[**NOTE:** We encourage you to look at the NCCN.org website yourself. But if you do, take the trouble to decipher the professional level recommendations. The statements designed for patients are over-simplified and lacking in detail.]

They also state the following:

"Clinical Trials: The NCCN recommends cancer patient participation in clinical trials as the gold standard for treatment.

"Cancer therapy selection, dosing, administration, and the management of related adverse events can be a complex process that should be handled by an experienced healthcare team.

Clinicians must choose and verify treatment options based on the individual patient; drug dose modifications and supportive care interventions should be administered accordingly. The cancer treatment regimens below may include both U.S. Food and Drug Administration-approved and unapproved indications/regimens. These regimens are provided only to supplement the latest treatment strategies.

"These Guidelines are a work in progress that may be refined as often as new significant data becomes available. The NCCN Guidelines® are a consensus statement of its authors regarding their views of currently accepted approaches to treatment. Any clinician seeking to apply or consult any NCCN Guidelines® is expected to use independent medical judgment in the context of individual clinical circumstances to determine any patient's care or treatment. The NCCN makes no warranties of any kind whatsoever regarding their content, use, or application and disclaims any responsibility for their application or use in any way."

BIBLIOGRAPHY

https://www.themossreport.com/bibliography.pdf

Complete list of sources cited throughout *The Moss Report - Cancer Treatment Guides*. 208pgs, and freely downloadable.

Made in United States
Orlando, FL
04 November 2026

90200491R00046